An Error in Judgement

The Politics of Medical Care in an Indian/White Community

Dara Culhane Speck

Talonbooks   •   Vancouver   •   1987

copyright © 1987 Dara Culhane Speck

published with the assistance of the Canada Council

Talonbooks
201 / 1019 East Cordova
Vancouver
British Columbia V6A 1M8
Canada

This book was typeset in Times by Pièce de Résistance Graphics, and printed and bound in Canada by Hignell Printing Ltd.

Third printing: June 1992

Canadian Cataloguing in Publication Data

Culhane Speck, Dara, 1950-
  An error in judgement

  Bibliography: p.
  ISBN 0-88922-246-0

  1. Indians of North America - British Columbia -
Alert Bay - Medical care - Case studies. 2.
Indians of North America - British Columbia -
Alert Bay - Medical care - Government policy -
Case studies. 3. Kwakiutl Indians - Medical care
- Case studies. 4. Kwakiutl Indians - Medical
care - Government policy - Case studies. I. Title.
RA418.3.C3C84 1987   362.1'08997071134   C87-091451-0

This book is dedicated to

PEARL ALFRED

backbone of a people

Contents

Acknowledgements

The mission of sociology is to understand the connections between history and biography, between social structure and personal histories, between public issues and private troubles.

— C. W. Mills

In acknowledging those who have made this book possible, first and foremost tribute must be paid to Renee Smith's family, whose courage led them to share their private troubles so that public issues could be illuminated. Without their strength, and their tireless devotion to their own community and to the Native community in Canada as a whole, this book would not have been written.

Second, respect must be accorded to the Native community in Alert Bay, particularly to those individuals who participated most actively in the events that are described in this book. It is their biographies that illustrate history, and their personal histories that reveal social structures. Without their enduring commitment to justice for Native peoples, and their inexhaustible dedication to making their community a better place to live in, the events I have documented would not have taken place.

Third, I wish to thank those who have practically assisted me in the researching and writing of this volume. First, thanks go to my husband, George Speck, Jr. In particular, the historical data, and the perspective from which it is presented, are drawn from his research into the historical "social character" of Kwakwaka'wakw[1] society. George has not only made these substantive contributions to the text, but he has also read and critiqued draft after draft of the manuscript. Furthermore, George was an active participant in the events described. After living together for fourteen years, and being students in the same faculty for four, we can no longer tell where his ideas end, and mine begin.

Another person with whom I shared the experiences recorded here most intimately, and with whom I have spent incalculable amounts of time in reflecting on these events, is my husband's cousin, Kelly Speck. We, too, have shared so many ideas and interpretations that it is futile to try to unravel them at this point.

One friend has been more help than she acknowledges. Miki Maeba and I met in 1976 when she began teaching at the T'ɫisalagi'lakw School in Alert Bay. Through countless hours of discussion over the years, we have helped each other gain insights and understandings neither of us could have found alone.

Professor Noel Dyck of Simon Fraser University introduced me to the concepts of tutelage and resistance in Indian/White relations, "bundles of beliefs" about Indians held by Canadians, and problems in Fourth World political representation. I would also like to thank Noel Dyck for the encouragement, guidance and patience he offered me during the writing of the original draft of this manuscript as my undergraduate honours thesis.

Journalists whose coverage of the events has been quoted at length are: Bill Smith, the *Victoria Daily Colonist*; Anne Roberts, the *Globe and Mail*; Andrea Maitland, the *Vancouver Sun*; and Bruce McLean, the *Vancouver Province*.

People who read earlier drafts of this manuscript and offered helpful advice are: Pearl Alfred, Dawna Ambers, Geri Ambers, John Bogardus, Eva Cook, Vera Cranmer, Dan Gillis, Fran Gillis, Professor Michael Jackson, Miki Maeba, Jane Mighton, Chavah Mintz, Elizabeth Nelson, Ethel Scow, Margaret Smith, Kelly Speck, Wedledi Speck, Renee Taylor, Gloria Cranmer Webster, Barbara Williamson.

Gary Fisher of Talonbooks gave me invaluable editorial assistance.

My mother, Claire, and my sister, Róisín, have, as always, been unfailing in their support and encouragement. My brother, Gary, generously provided professional legal advice.

And, last but by no means least, my children, Carey and Lori Speck, have been patient and helpful throughout, and are my greatest source of inspiration. This book is written for them, and for their generation, in the hope that by learning from history they may be better able to shape the future.

Royalties from the sale of this book will be divided equally between the author and the *Renee Smith Memorial Health Care Fund*.

Foreword

1987 will no doubt go down in the history books of Canada as the year in which Quebec was brought back into the fold of Confederation. Following the Meech Lake Accord, the Prime Minister and the provincial premiers agreed to a constitutional amendment which entrenches the rights of Quebec as a distinct society. But what probably will not be recorded in the history books is that in 1987 the same Prime Minister and provincial premiers failed to reach an accord to entrench in the Constitution the rights of Native people to self-government. Provincial concerns about the vagueness of the constitutional language, raised to defeat entrenchment of Native peoples' "right to self-government," were put aside when it came to recognition of Quebec's rights as "a distinct society." Concerns as to the dire consequences for the future of Canada in not reaching an accord with Quebec led to a marathon all-night session by the First Ministers to hammer out a consensus. By contrast, at the Conference on Native Rights no such alarms were raised and the meetings concluded at the end of a working day without even a commitment to further constitutional talks.

Yet, in the enormous publicity that has attended the Meech Lake Accord hardly anyone (apart from Native people) has commented on the perversity and the paradox of acknowledging the constitutional significance and entrenching the constitutional distinctiveness of Quebec within Confederation, based on 400 years of history in North America, while refusing to acknowledge and recognize the significance of Native peoples' distinctive place in that same Confederation based on over 10,000 years of their history on this continent.

The failure to even recognize, let alone redress, this paradox is not rooted in the politics of liberal democracy (there are more Quebecois than Native people and they carry more political clout) but in the politics of racism and colonialism. It is rooted in the continuing failure of Canadians to accept Native peoples as equals and contemporaries. The dark legacy of superiorist attitudes and policies directed at Native peoples explains not only the constitutional events of 1987, it lies at the heart of Dara Culhane Speck's *An Error In Judgement*.

An Error in Judgement is based on an event in the life of an Indian community in 1979—the death of an eleven-year-old girl from an undiagnosed ruptured appendix—which on the surface of things would seem to be a human tragedy belonging to the personal history of the child's family and of legal significance only in terms of the civil liability of the physician involved. However, as the political and historical overlays of this event are peeled back, we come to see that this is more than the stuff of personal suffering and individual responsibility. Informed by a historical understanding of the relationship between Indians and Whites as it has evolved over the last century in Alert Bay (and other Canadian frontiers of colonial expansion), we are made to realize that the events of 1979 are not an exception to, but a reflection of, underlying attitudes towards Indians. This story involves not simply matters of individual, but collective rights and responsibilities. We are made aware of the ways in which in the last 100 years there has been a systematic undermining of Native peoples' ability to determine the shape of their own lives, a progressive and debilitating draining of their strength by a succession of missionaries, Indian Agents, health care professionals and child care workers, whose work has been informed by a common mandate to bring the benefits of a "civilized" society to those who are seen to exist at an earlier stage of evolutionary development.

The exploration of the historical patterns of colonialism in British Columbia is not uncharted territory. Historians, political scientists, anthropologists and legal scholars have mined the archival record. *An Error in Judgement* brings to this body of work a striking contemporary relevance. We read the words of nineteenth-century missionaries and Indian Agents and find their mirror images a century later, the idiom a little different but the superiorist assumptions still unmistakable. What is also new and distinctive about *An Error in Judgement* is that the task of identifying the root causes of the poor health of Native people in Alert Bay and the struggle of Native people to change that grim reality by regaining control over their lives, is traced through the words of the Indian community itself. Woven into the fabric of the book are the statements of Native people at a series of provincial and federal inquests, hearings and inquiries triggered by the death of a child but culminating in a searing indictment of Indian policy in Canada.

What we find in *An Error in Judgement*, therefore, is not another sociological study coined in the academy, but an authentic account of the Indian experience of colonialism, documented through the public record, informed by a grass-roots understanding of an Indian community, given perspective with a scholarly review of history, and charged with an activist's commitment to changing political and social realities.

We are given in *An Error in Judgement* an opportunity to understand the roots of racism in Canada from the inside out. There will be no Meech Lake Accord for Native people and no Confederation founded on justice and respect for the rights of Native people until these roots are acknowledged and racism is eradicated. It is works like *An Error in Judgement*, rather than their briefing books, that the Prime Minister and the premiers should read when they next meet with the Native peoples of Canada.

Professor Michael Jackson
Faculty of Law, University of British Columbia

Introduction

This is a story about the town of Alert Bay and its experiences during a prolonged crisis which spanned an eighteen-month period: January 1979-June 1980. Alert Bay is a small town on British Columbia's northwest coast, situated on Cormorant Island adjacent to the northeastern end of Vancouver Island. In 1979-80, Alert Bay supported a population of approximately fifteen hundred people, about nine hundred of whom were Indians[1] of the Kwakwaka'wakw, while the remaining six hundred were non-Indians, primarily Euro-Canadian Whites. This crisis began with the death of an eleven-year-old child, Renee Smith, from acute appendicitis, in the local hospital.

Appendicitis is a very common ailment, especially among young people of Renee's age. It is an ailment from which, statistics show, children rarely die nowadays. But, in 1979, an eleven-year-old Native girl complaining of severe abdominal pain, diarrhea, and nausea entered a modern, well-equipped hospital in British Columbia and died, four days later, from a ruptured appendix.

"Why did Renee Smith die?" This question was asked over and over again during the eighteen months that followed Renee's death. Answers were offered by such diverse groups as Renee's family and her community; the doctor who attended her, Jack Pickup; the St. George's Hospital staff; a Coroner's Inquest; the B.C. College of Physicians and Surgeons, the governing body of the British Columbia medical profession; an inquiry sponsored by the B.C. Ministry of Health; an inquiry conducted by a representative of the Anglican Church of Canada; members of the legal profession; the press; Native and non-Native political organizations; and, finally, in May of 1980, a commission of inquiry sponsored by the federal Minister of National Health and Welfare. In the search for an answer to this question, the foundations of a century-old relationship between an indigenous community, colonial settlers, professionals, and a modern, liberal, democratic state were publicly and dramatically illustrated, debated, criticized and challenged.

This story, then, is really about two groups of people, Natives and non-Natives, inextricably tied together in a network of complex relationships which have developed over a period of approximately 100 years, since the beginning of intensive European settlement on the British Columbia coast. It is also a story about an episode in the struggle to change these relationships, a struggle which is as old as the town of Alert Bay itself.

The central core of this book is a documentary record of these events. All sources are acknowledged and referenced, and all may be found within the public record. As such, the data are available to any other researcher who may wish to investigate, or verify, the events recorded here. I have made extensive use of verbatim quotations throughout this book, the sources of which may also be found within the public record. I began to employ this technique as a matter of principle in that I wished to allow people to speak for themselves as much as possible. I soon found, however, that such a technique was a matter of necessity in relaying this particular story, because what people say is inseparable from how they say it. As well as providing readers with an opportunity to respond directly to the participants' own expressions of opinion and emotion, I hope this mode of presentation will further serve to allow readers to criticize, analyze and form their own opinions on the basis of this documentation.

Therefore, this is a true story. It is not, however, an unbiased one. There are many, I know, who are as familiar with the events documented here as I am, who will read this account and say "That's not the way it was at all." But I am confident that there are none who could say "That's not what happened."

During the time of the crisis, and for several years before it reached its peak, I lived in the Native community, and I took an active part in the events which form the basis of this story. The main bias I would expect a critical reader to point out is that this account is more sympathetic to the Native community than to either the local White community, or the agencies outside Alert Bay that played a role in this story. This is a bias that I think arises from my personal history, as well as from the facts of the case at hand, and I shall endeavour to set out the factors that I believe influence my point of view, and that, as such, have acted as filters to my observation, recording, and interpretation of the experiences described here.

I was born in 1950, the child of a "mixed" marriage. My mother is a Jewish woman from Montreal, the daughter of Eastern European immigrants. My father is an Irishman from Dublin, the son of Catholic Nationalists. I spent my early childhood in Vancouver, Quebec and the Republic of Ireland. In 1960, at the age of ten, I returned with my mother to Montreal, where I lived until 1969. My parents were political activists in whose lives public struggles for social justice always played a central role. While both came from middle class families, they paid the price exacted of many activists of their day and did not establish prestigious careers or lucrative incomes. While I was growing up, our family's main source of support, and therefore the basis of our material standard of living, was my mother's earnings from secretarial work. I became aware early in life of both the narrow-minded ethnocentrism of my parents' respective families, and of the insidious class snobbery and ethnic chauvinism which is so integral a part of Canadian, and British, society. My involvement as a young adult in political and cultural movements during the 1960s and 1970s also contributed to the way in which I viewed a community like Alert Bay when I moved there in my early twenties.

Most relevant to my understanding of the particular events this book describes, however, was my social location within Alert Bay. The terms "Indian" and "White," in Alert Bay, define categories of people of which a part of the definition includes racial/ethnic origins recognized by society as a whole, while the other part of the definition refers to a given individual's local situation. I am a White woman, married to an Indian man, and we have two children. I lived on the reserve for eight years and have been closely connected to it, through bonds of family and friendship, for a total of fourteen years. I am, therefore, not an Indian, but I am part of the Indian community. I am white, but I am not a part of the White community. This is not always an easy or a comfortable position to be in, but it is one which I hope has allowed me to gain insights and understandings of the White community which come from an "it takes one to know one" perspective. My understandings of the Indian community come from my observations and experiences of living within that community and being forced, sometimes painfully, to see things from their perspective.

While in Alert Bay, I worked as a mother of two children, as a waitress in the bars, as a taxi driver, as a community development worker employed by the Nimpkish Band Council, as a "trainee," and as a vocational instructor. My husband and many of his close relatives were actively involved, during the 1970s, in Indian political organizations and movements at local, regional and provincial levels and in band administration. I participated in much of this activity including the organizing of a food co-op, a Land Claims Committee, and an independent band-operated school on reserve. The 1970s were years of particular tension between the sector of the Indian community with which I was involved, and local non-Indians, and provincial and federal governments. As such, my informal interaction throughout these years was almost exclusively with members of the Indian community, and with non-Indians who were peripheral to both the Indian and the White communities.

Crises have a way of illuminating, intensifying, and throwing into sharp relief, underlying structures that shape relationships between people and that are often blurred in the course of everyday life. Trying to understand the relationship between Native communities and Canadian society as a whole has brought me face to face with the most fundamental contradictions in Canadian society. I have never been able to see the world in quite the same way since I became a part of the Indian community in Alert Bay. Many of us who experienced and tried to make sense of the crisis documented here have not been able to see our place in the world in quite the same way since.

My explicit objective has been to present this story as it was experienced and understood by people in the Native community, and particularly by the activists within that community. This is a point of view that, I have found, is rarely heard from, documented, accepted as credible at face value, or treated seriously. I believe, therefore, that the bias in this book is predominantly one that views the attitudes and actions of non-Indians from a perspective that is, to some extent, conditioned by the personal factors outlined above, but is also that of the people in the Native community who were most actively involved in the events described here. These people have read an earlier draft of the manuscript, and offered suggestions and criticisms which I have tried to incorporate into the book. These readers have told me that the text accurately represents their memories of the specific events. Since I lived the events documented here, and have reflected on them with other participants during countless hours of discussion in the years since 1979, I cannot say that the general impressions, interpretations, or analyses offered here are "mine." Nevertheless, I have written this book; I have told the story from my point of view; and I take full responsibility for it.

I have tried to look fairly at the "other side," that is, at sectors of the non-Indian community in Alert Bay, and the institutions and government ministries outside of the community that became involved in the crisis, with whom I had, and still have, limited contact. I have also endeavoured to look critically at myself and "my side." To this end, I have drawn on a wide range of sources, including published material pertaining to the actual events described, correspondence, newspaper articles, my personal diaries, and social science literature on the topics covered by this book. I have not, however, personally consulted with, nor provided copies of manuscript drafts to, the "other side." Another point which should be taken into consideration in this regard is that throughout the process described in this book, the Indian community and its allies relied for support upon public opinion, while the "other side" placed its faith in official channels and presented its case in forums whose proceedings are not made available to the public. Available information therefore reflects this difference in strategies.

All this having been said, I would add that I do not think that we live in the "best of all possible worlds." The issues upon which this story is based demand(ed) that sides be chosen, and I have no regrets about which side I was (am) on. For this I offer no apologies.

Alert Bay is, in many ways, a unique place. As in so many island communities, it often feels to those who live there as though their experiences are unconnected to anything or anyone else in the universe. However, no woman or man is an island, and no island floats freely in time, or in physical, social or political space. I have tried, therefore, to surround this particular story about unique individuals in one place, during a specific period of time, with context. I have attempted to follow connections from the island and its people to the "outside," as these connections became visible during the course of events. I then traced these connections to their sources and to the contexts that, in turn, gave rise to them.

We are educated to think of the world, and our lives, as being divided into separate and distinct compartments, each of which can be studied and understood in isolation from the other. We describe our physical environment as "geography"; our past as "history"; our customs, attitudes and beliefs as "culture." We divide our present into "personal life," "family life," "working life," "political life." Yet each day, as each of us goes about the business of living, we experience the interrelatedness—the synthetic totality—of all of these spheres that we so neatly cut up and package in their own little boxes and university faculties.

When non-Indians think about Indians and "Indian problems," these too are itemized and each is considered separately from the others. There are "land questions," "legislative problems," "legal issues," and "health problems." There are issues like "racism," "culture," and "cross-cultural communication" to be taken account of. When these questions are examined closely, however, and/or when Indian people themselves are listened to attentively and with open minds, it becomes very clear that questions concerning land, economy, culture and health must be conceptualized as one, and not four, issues. So it is too that in order to understand how the death of one little girl, in one little town, could attract so much attention, and cause so much concern, to both local townspeople and various levels of government in a nation state, it is necessary to understand the whole context in which this event was enmeshed.

The book begins, in Chapters 1, 2 and 3, with a description of Renee Smith's death and the events that precipitated the crisis following this tragedy. Chief Roy Cranmer, of the Nimpkish Indian Band, began his address to the federal Inquiry in which this crisis culminated in March 1980 with the words, "We hope to show to you, Mr. Commissioner, and to the Canadian public, that the problems we face here to-day go far beyond the practices of one local doctor. They date back 100 years, to the way of thinking that characterizes non-Indian attitudes to Indian people." Accordingly, the first connections I have drawn are those of historical time and space.

Chapter 4 begins with a glimpse of Kwakwaka'wakw society before the arrival of Europeans on the British Columbia coast, briefly explains the role of shamans and healers within that society, and describes the initial contacts between the Kwakwaka'wakw and European fur traders. This chapter then travels across both time and space to nineteenth-century Britain—to the origins of the European colonists who settled in the Kwakwaka'wakw area, and particularly to the origins of their "way of thinking" about Indian people. Finally, Chapter 4 outlines the relationship between Indians and non-Indians as it has developed in Alert Bay over the past 100 years, and ends with a description of the social, economic and political structures of Alert Bay's two communities, the relationships between their members, and the forces which shaped their respective responses to Renee Smith's death in 1979.

Chapter 5 documents the inquest that was held into her death, and through the testimonies of witnesses, the strategies of lawyers, and the responses of the provincial and national press and public opinion, we are given further insights into the historical and contemporary connections between the island and the society which surrounds and dominates it, and how these connections were experienced by ordinary people in a small reserve community. Chapter 6 describes the actions of local people in response to the inquest jury's alarming verdict.

Chapter 7 once again leaves Cormorant Island and follows connections through social and political space. In this chapter the responses to the crisis by the provincial government of British Columbia, the medical profession, and the federal government of Canada are explored and analyzed. The influence of expert opinion and current professional approaches to Native health and health care are examined in this context, as well as the problems which arise from the self-policing nature of the medical profession. The effect of legal and legislative mandates, federal/provincial jurisdictional disputes and government policies in the field of Native health care, are viewed from the perspective of both their impact on the crisis in Alert Bay, and their relevance to the delivery of health care to Native peoples across Canada.

Chapter 8 returns once again to Cormorant Island, specifically to the Native community, and traces the impact of the external responses documented in Chapter 7 on relationships within that community. This chapter describes how local politicians and community activists debated various strategies to resolve the crisis; how they defined their relationship to provincial and national Native organizations; and how they coped with the internal conflicts and factionalism the crisis had produced.

Chapters 9 and 10 describe two incidents that took place in this community during the fall of 1979 and the early winter of 1980, and which give credence to the old adage: "truth is stranger than fiction." These chapters introduce two unique individuals who never knew each other, but whom history and

18

circumstance brought to one place at one time and thus connected one to the other.

Chapter 11 documents the federal inquiry which ostensibly brought the crisis to a close. In the context of this inquiry, all the key players—local people, health care professionals, government representatives and Native politicians—come together in an intense power struggle within a single forum. From this explosion of bitterness, emotion, frustration, and competing interpretations, emerges a "solution" which embodies the heart of the crisis itself.

Chapter 12 returns to the Alert Bay of 1895. The end of the story brings us back to its beginning.

The Epilogue visits Cormorant Island three years after the crisis abated, and briefly sketches the ongoing effects of its aftermath.

As with the observations and interpretations of the specific occurrences recounted here, my perception of meaningful connections is also influenced by both personal and social factors. In 1982, approximately two years after this story came to an end, at the age of thirty-two, I began to attend Simon Fraser University, from where I graduated in 1985 with an honours degree in Sociology and Anthropology. I am now in my third year of a Ph.D. program in Anthropology and Sociology at the University of British Columbia. Therefore, the rendition which I now offer, and the perspective from which I now view these events, is influenced (or, some would say, distorted) by a distance of time—eight years—between the events and this writing; and by a distance of perception—a university degree in social science. These differences in perception are represented first by the subjective interpretation of the story itself, which is based on points of view and feelings I recorded in my personal journals, kept at the time of the events, and gleaned from memory and subsequent conversations. Second, the contextual material is drawn from historical documentation, and from data, analyses, comparisons and generalizations found within the literature of social science, particularly history and anthropology.

Finally, and, I believe, most importantly, I must answer the question that must be answered by any author: Why write this book?

Although this is a question I have asked myself, and others, for many years now, the decision to do so has not been one that I have made lightly. The events recorded here were extremely painful for many people to live through, and although it is now eight years later, the wounds still open easily. Renee's family lost a precious child. An entire town had to come to terms with itself and with the consequences of circumstances and relationships that most townspeople had had little role in creating. Everyone on Cormorant Island was compelled to face themselves and each other with a brutal honesty, the likes of which most people have the luxury of being able to avoid during the course of an ordinary lifetime. Therefore, I know there are people who will feel that nothing good can come out of setting it all down in a book like this, stirring up uncomfortable memories, and preventing people from forgetting. There will be people in Alert Bay who will resent the privacy of their little town being so intruded upon by a permanent record such as this. However, there are circumstances in which silence becomes a weapon which perpetuates injustice, and privacy a shield that allows the powerful to abuse their positions. I decided now, as the participants in these events decided in 1979, that this was such a case.

The situation in Alert Bay is not unique, and neither is Dr. Pickup. This book is not an attack on one individual man who is, like all of us, only a fallible human being. Rather, it is a critique of a system of relationships between people which has ramifications beyond the boundaries of Cormorant Island. Similar situations arise over and over again in hundreds of Native communities across Canada, not only in the sphere of medical care but in education, economic development, land rights, social welfare, law enforcement and local government. Native people are involved in seeking ways and means to change these institutions, and the relationships embodied in them, in positive and productive ways. It is my hope that by reading this account of our experiences in Alert Bay, people will gain insights into this process that will help to advance this movement.

When I circulated an early draft of this book to the people in Alert Bay who participated in these experiences, and asked them if they thought it should be published, everyone, without exception, said "Yes. Publish it. People should know about this." People outside of Alert Bay, to whom I also circulated an early draft, said the same thing. I have thought a lot about this response—this desire to make people see, to make people understand, to make people change. It was this that spurred us and sustained us through the eighteen months of the crisis. This was the motivation that drove me to produce this book.

It is a desire that, if logical, must be based, first of all, on the assumption that if the less powerful in our society had greater knowledge and understanding of the people and structures which keep them dependent and subordinate, they would be better able to effect change. On the other hand, it is a desire that also reflects the hope that if people who abuse their power over others knew and understood the depth of the human pain they inflict, they would change.

Therefore it is, I believe, in the sharing of experiences such as the ones described in this book, where hope for the future lies. This story itself does not offer much encouragement in this regard. People were told, and told again, and they did not change. Structures which maintain and perpetuate unequal and unjust relationships were challenged, and challenged again, and they did not change. Many of the injured parties could not find within themselves, or within the conditions under which they live, the will, the strength, or the opportunity, to sustain a prolonged struggle. This story does not have a happy ending. But if the recounting of it can contribute in some way to the development of a more just relationship between Indians and non-Indians in Canada, then it will have been worth telling.

> *The important thing is to pull yourself up by the roots of your own hair*
> *To turn yourself inside out, and see the whole world with fresh eyes.*
> —Jean Paul Marat

These are the reasons why I have written this book.

NOTES:

The Kwakwaka'wakw (Kwa'kwala-speaking peoples) have been classified as a single entity under the collective label "Kwakiutl" by anthropologists, and "Kwawkewlths" by government administrators. In fact, however, there were, before the arrival of Europeans, approximately eighteen relatively autonomous bands of people who spoke the same language but who lived in different locales and had different names for themselves. Anthropologists claim that there were eight local clusters of neighbouring bands and that all eighteen bands had relationships with each other, and with other linguistic groups up and down the coast and the mainland, based on trade and inter-marriage. In recent years, members of the various Kwakwaka'wakw bands have been involved in the process of reclaiming their history and correcting various public versions of it. As part of this movement, they have begun to refer to themselves as the Kwakwaka'wakw to more accurately reflect the historical and contemporary reality of their socio-political structure.

[1]The labelling of North and South American Indigenous peoples as "Indians" results from the error made by Christopher Columbus who believed, when he landed on the shores of the Americas in 1492, that he had reached India. The term not only ignores the existence on these continents, prior to European colonization, of many varied and autonomous aboriginal nations, but also carries with it many negative connotations which arise from the colonial experience. As such, many indigenous peoples prefer to be known by the name which denotes their particular national origin or by the more correct general term "Native." In unself-conscious everyday discourse, however, people in Alert Bay refer to themselves and others by all three labels: "Kwakiutl or Kwakwaka'wakw," "Native" and "Indian" according to the specific context in which the term is being used. Believing that language both *reflects and reinforces* social reality, and in the interests of accuracy, I have tried to *reflect* this everyday use pattern in the text, while not intending to *reinforce* the negative connotations which are connected with the term "Indian."

CHAPTER 1

Renee Bernice Smith

Alert Bay, B.C.
January 1979

Arthur Dick, Sr. is a successful man by anyone's standards. In 1979 he owned
two large seine boats, each employing five men fishing salmon and herring
off British Columbia's west coast. A member of the Nimpkish Indian Band
situated at Alert Bay, Mr. Dick had served intermittently on the elected Band
Council of his reserve community for many years; he had been an active member
of the Native Brotherhood of British Columbia, an organization formed in 1931
to lobby for improvements in opportunities for B.C. Indians; and he was a
high-ranking chief and host of many lavish and well-attended potlatches. Coming
from a big family himself, he had married a woman from a large and prestigious
local family and together they had raised seven children: six daughters and a son.

Arthur Dick's daughters—"the Dick girls," as they are known locally—are
a force to be reckoned with. Exuberant, affectionate and ferociously loyal allies,
they can be equally formidable enemies. The girls, their mother and their children
could be seen daily spilling out of a big car, pick-up truck or station wagon
as they drove up and down the town's main road shopping together, collecting
mail together, picking kids up from school together, and organizing the endless
round of birthday parties, showers, anniversary dinners, weddings, funerals,
and potlatches around which the social life of a big family revolves.

The Dick girls form part of that brigade of women who keep the Native
community going. It is these women who sit on the band committees concerned
with local education, social and health services and cultural revival and

development. They organize the athletic clubs, the soccer tournaments, the dances, and the fund-raising raffles, bake sales and pot-luck dinners. Most of the men in the village, like Mr. Dick's only son, Arthur Dick, Jr., concentrate on fishing, which, until the recent decline in the industry, took them away from home for several months at a time throughout the year. It is the men who are most often Band Councillors and/or who become involved in the Native Brotherhood.

The 1978 salmon season had been lucrative for some of Alert Bay's commercial fishermen, including Arthur Dick, Sr., who was among those who could boast of having been a "highliner" that year. In January of 1979, when his grandchildren had returned to school after the Christmas holidays, Mr. Dick, Mrs. Dick, four of their daughters, two sons-in-law, and his son and daughter-in-law left to spend a week in Reno to celebrate their good fortune and to take a break before herring fishing began in February.

His daughter Margaret and her husband, Richard Smith, had never travelled this far from home before and they were especially excited about the trip.

The Nimpkish Indian Reserve, called "The Village," occupies half of five-mile long, half-mile wide Cormorant Island, which lies midway between Vancouver Island and the B.C. mainland, surrounded by the waters of Johnstone Strait. Approximately 700 of the 1000 members of the Nimpkish Indian Band live there so it was easy for Margaret and Richard to find a babysitter from among their extended family to look after their two children for them while they were away in Reno.

Richard's brother, Leonard, moved into Margaret and Richard's home to take charge of Renee, aged eleven and Richard Jr., aged six and on Thursday, January 11, 1979, an elated entourage left Alert Bay for the bright lights of Reno.

Renee and Richard Jr. both had sniffles and sore throats when Margaret and Richard left and when, by Saturday, their colds appeared to be getting worse, Leonard opted for a "better safe than sorry" strategy and took both children to see Dr. Harold J. "Jack" Pickup, the island's sole medical practitioner. Dr. Pickup prescribed cough medicine and pills to be taken every four hours.

Leonard kept his charges home from school on Monday but by Tuesday their colds had cleared up and they went back to school. On Wednesday Renee complained to Leonard that her stomach hurt and throughout the day she was troubled by vomiting and diarrhea. The medicine prescribed on Saturday was finished so Leonard decided to take her back to the doctor. The doctor is away on Wednesdays and his clinic is closed all day so Leonard called the hospital and explained his niece's symptoms to a nurse, telling her that he was especially worried because now she seemed to be having bad stomach pains. The nurse told him to bring her down to the hospital so they could take a look at her.

St. George's Hospital is a white, wooden, blue-trimmed building whose grounds encompass a doctor's clinic and offices as well as a nurse's residence and a small chapel. The hospital is situated on the island's main road, and is flanked on one side by the Indian graveyard with its tall, cedar totem poles and on the other by the doctor's British-style home with its flower garden, shrubbery, and greenhouse. The hospital complex, the doctor's home and the Indian graveyard are all located on the southern half of Cormorant Island, designated as the Municipality of Alert Bay, and referred to locally as "The White End." Indians point to the location of their graveyard in the middle of the municipality as evidence that every time a surveyor shows up in town, the reserve gets smaller and the municipality larger.

Renee was having trouble standing up straight and it was so painful for her to move at all that Leonard had to help her out of the cab and support her with his arm as they walked into St. George's. At the hospital Renee and her uncle were seen by a young woman who had nursed since 1974 when she completed training in her native Philippines. After having him sign some forms and pay the two-dollar out-patient fee, the nurse asked Leonard to wait outside while she took Renee into a private examining room. She noted Renee's symptoms: nausea, diarrhea and severe abdominal pain, and asked Renee to lie down so she could examine her. A distraught Renee pushed the nurse's hand away and said she didn't want to be examined. The nurse then called the doctor at his home next door and explained the girl's symptoms. Dr. Pickup told her to admit Renee for observation. The nurse relayed this advice to Renee who responded, crying, "I don't have to stay in your damned hospital! Just give me a pain killer! I'm in pain!" The nurse placed a second call to Dr. Pickup and reported Renee's refusal. Dr. Pickup prescribed 642s for pain and suggested that Leonard be told to bring Renee back the next day if her condition had not improved. The nurse reported this information to Renee, handed her an envelope containing eight Darvon-N capsules and sent her and her uncle on their way.

Despite the medication, Renee's symptoms worsened and the next morning— Thursday, January 18th—Leonard phoned the doctor's office and explained to the receptionist, Mrs. Pickup, that Renee was still throwing up, still in pain and only drinking apple juice. Mrs. Pickup gave him an appointment for 4:30 p.m. that day. When they arrived, Dr. Pickup X-rayed Renee's chest and told Leonard that Renee "had to have an operation right away." Leonard agreed to hospitalization but said he didn't think he could give consent for an operation until he had contacted Renee's vacationing parents.

"I can't wait that long," Dr. Pickup cautioned. Leonard replied that he didn't think he had the legal right to authorize an operation and would try to contact Margaret and Richard immediately. At 5:20 p.m. Leonard pushed his niece, in a wheelchair, from the doctor's office to the admitting desk in the adjoining hospital. A nurse hastily completed admitting procedures, copied Dr. Pickup's diagnosis of "acute abdomen" onto a patient chart, noted that Renee appeared "pale, anxious and in considerable pain" and gave Leonard a form to sign, explaining that it was a routine admitting form. Guessing at Renee's weight in order to determine appropriate dosages, the admitting nurse began to administer the four different drugs the doctor had ordered to combat pain, nausea, infection and fever.

After seeing his niece settled in a hospital bed, Leonard returned home to contact Renee's parents and to notify other relatives. Once Renee's condition was known, female relatives who worked as kitchen help and cleaning women in the hospital checked in on Renee whenever they had a break, while other relatives took turns sitting by her bedside round the clock, comforting her, seeing to her needs, reporting their observations of her condition to the nurses, and questioning the doctor when he arrived to make his rounds. Such vigils are common practice among Alert Bay area Indians when a family member, particularly a child, is hospitalized with a serious ailment.

Leonard reached his brother, Richard, in Reno on Thursday evening, January 18th. The entire Dick family group cut their holiday short, rearranged plane reservations as quickly as possible, and returned to Alert Bay on the evening of Friday, January 19th. Margaret's sister, Ethel Scow, had taken her annual holiday leave from her job as receptionist at the Indian Health Office to go to Reno with her family. On February 3, 1979, two weeks after Renee was first hospitalized, Ethel wrote a detailed account of the time she had spent with Renee at St. George's, beginning with the family's return to Alert Bay and their arrival at the hospital on Friday night.

Ethel:

Friday, January 19, 1979

I arrived at the hospital at 9:40 p.m. with her [Renee's] parents... my sister Vera Cranmer and a cousin, was sitting with her when we arrived. Only the parents were allowed into her room at first....Vera told me the Doctor told her that Renee had the worst case of the flu, and that it affected Children more, this is why she got so sick, but she was improving. I went in to see Renee for a few minutes, and told her I'd come and sit with her in the morning. I was very upset to see her in that condition.

Saturday, January 20th, 1979

I arrived at the hospital at around 9:40 a.m. Renee seemed a lot better to me in appearance. I asked Margaret, my sister, if she spoke to the Doctor the night before and he told her he thought it was her appendix. But he didn't think he needed to operate, because she had improved considerably, and there was nothing to worry about. I asked her if Renee slept at all through the night, and she said that she was very restless, and slept little. I told Margaret I would sit with Renee so her and Richard could get some sleep.

I noticed that her heart was beating rapidly. When looking at Renee, it was quite noticeable, just in between her collar bone and neck, the skin there was moving rapidly. This was like that the evening before, I also noticed.

A nurse came into her room to give her pills to take. Renee threw this all up later.

Another nurse came into her room and told me to make sure she drank a lot of juice, and to keep moving her arms and legs around. She also said to make her take deep breaths in order to exercise her lungs. This was to help prevent her from getting pneumonia. Renee was doing this all that time I sat with her and it was quite painful for her to do. I asked her if she felt any better, she said yes, just her pains in her stomach.

A nurse came later to take her temperature and I asked her what it was, and she said 37.6 degrees. I then asked her what was normal, she said 36 degrees. I was happy to hear that.

Ethel remained at the hospital throughout the day. She encouraged Renee to do the exercises the nurse had recommended, fed her, and then changed her nightgown and linen as Renee repeatedly vomited whatever she ingested. Ethel reported each incident to the nurses, to the steady stream of relatives who visited and to the doctor who examined the child's still painful abdomen twice that day.
Ethel:

Renee said she wanted to sit up, which she did for about a minute. She laid back down, and then threw up...I went and got a nurse and it was the Head Nurse. She helped her out of bed and moved her to a chair to sit on while her bedding got changed. The nurse then adjusted her bed to a sitting position. She helped Renee back to bed and this was again a very painful thing for her to do. I told the Head Nurse that Renee was throwing up a lot, and that I had to keep changing her nightgown and emptying out her emesis basin.

Dr. Pickup came to examine her around 11:00 a.m. He had a stethoscope with him and he felt around her stomach pressing it, and this caused a lot of pain for Renee. He then listened to her heart. I asked him how she was and he told me she was improving and he seemed pleased that she was up for a few minutes. I told him about her being so nauseated, and asked him if there was anything he could do for her about this.

The Doctor prescribed anti-nausea medication and assured the family that Renee would be fine.
Ethel:

One of the nurses came in and gave Renee a pill to help prevent her nausea. She brought this up shortly after.

At noon her lunch tray was brought to her. I fed her some soup, gave her a bit of juice and I fed her a bit of jello. One of the nurses came and told me to make sure she had a bit to eat. I told her I had already given her a little bit of everything on her tray. About 20 minutes later Renee brought all this up and I again changed her nightgown. Dr. Pickup came in to check her again. He did the same thing he did that morning, feeling around her stomach, and she screamed out saying that it hurts.

At 2:00 p.m. Margaret came back and I told her of what was happening that morning. Mum came to visit and she seemed pleased that Renee looked a lot better, compared to the evening before. Dad was also there. A nurse came in again to take her temperature and I asked her what it was and she said 38 degrees. I mentioned to her again that Renee was still throwing up. One of the nurses came and gave her a needle. We were asked to leave the room. When we went back to Renee's room my other sister Eva was there. She stayed about half an hour and then went to do her grocery shopping with Mum and Margaret. I told her that I would sit with Renee until she got back. A different nurse came to take Renee's temperature. I asked her what it was but she wouldn't tell me, because I wasn't the parent of her.

Sunday, January 21, 1979

I arrived at the hospital at 2:00 p.m.. Renee was still throwing up, and still very restless. Mum and Dad arrived shortly after I got there. Dad was very concerned about her so he left to go and inquire about her condition. He spoke to the Head Nurse. He expressed his concern over her, and he wanted her to be transferred to a hospital in Vancouver. The nurse told him she was improving. Later on the Head Nurse brought in a suppository, to prevent Renee from throwing up. Renee did not like the idea, but we reassured her that she would feel so much better and so she agreed. We stood outside her room and could hear Renee saying that it hurt.

At 5:45 p.m. the doctor came to examine her again and I asked him why she was still throwing up and he said that it wasn't on her chart. I told him that the two days that I've been with Renee thats all she's been doing. He then replied again that it wasn't on her chart. I got quite annoyed with him and I said you mean to tell me that every time she threw up, that I was to report it to the nurse? Well, I said, that is what we have been doing. We had been reporting everything to the nurses all along.

At 6:45 p.m. the admitting nurse came to check on Renee and she told me she was going to check with the doctor to see if she could start an intravenous on her. She told me she couldn't understand why they didn't start it yesterday.

At 7:00 p.m. Renee got two of her cousins visiting her, and she was happy to see them. I left the hospital then. I stopped by the T.V. room to talk to Renee's father. Richard had come to sit with her for the night and I told him to make sure to let the nurses know if she kept throwing up because the doctor didn't seem to believe me when I was telling him. I told him I would be back around 8:30 in the morning to replace him.

Monday, January 22, 1979

When I came the next morning Richard told me that Renee had severe pains in her stomach during the night. She wanted her Mum so I went to call Margaret and she had to make arrangements first so Richard stayed until she got there.

Throughout the morning, Renee's condition deteriorated.
Ethel:

One of the Philippine nurses came with a wheel chair to take her for X-rays. Renee kept on screaming, saying that her stomach hurt. I helped the nurse move her, and carried the I.V. Two X-rays were taken of her, one lying down and one standing up. All during the X-rays she cried out, saying her stomach hurt. The Nurse and I brought her back to her room, and she kept crying out, "My stomach! It hurts!" I felt so bad. I was almost in tears, seeing her that way.

A lab technician came and got two vials of blood from Renee's arm. I questioned her on what they were for, and she said one was to test her blood count, and the other, I couldn't understand because of her Philippine accent.

Another nurse came in to give Renee more needles. I told her the nurse had told me the night before that everything was going to come from the I.V. because poor Renee's rear end was so sore from all those needles she was getting. The nurse told me that she only took orders from the Doctor.

The doctor came by around 11:00 a.m. again and checked her. I asked him what her X-rays showed and he said she was full of gas, that this was the reason why she was in so much pain. He said he would order an enema. I then questioned him on the results of her blood test and he said he hadn't gotten the results of it and that it still could be her appendix. "I don't know, it still could be that," he said. Then he shrugged his shoulders and left the room. Later on they gave her a nasal gastric tube to relieve the gas. I asked the nurse how long the tubes were going to be in and she said a couple of days, maybe even a week. I said that one of the other nurses told me it was only going to be for a couple of hours. "Well it's like a plugged up sink," she told me. "You have to clear the contents out before it will start to work again."

At 2:00 p.m. Mum arrived, and she was quite concerned about Renee's condition. She also noticed that she wasn't getting any better. She told me to go and talk to the Nurse or Doctor about transferring her down to Vancouver. When I did that I was told that we couldn't see the doctor until 4:30—after his clinic hours. I went back to Renee's room and told Margaret and Mum that and then I asked Margaret if she would like Eva to come down so that they could both go and see the doctor together because Eva is not shy like Margaret is. Margaret said yes so I went and phoned Eva to come down and see about getting Renee transferred out. I told Margaret to make sure they asked for the Air Sea Rescue plane to come for Renee and I told her to see if she could go to St. Paul's instead of the Vancouver General. Then I left to go and pick up a few groceries for supper. I told Margaret I would go home and cook something for her to eat because she hadn't eaten all day.

I phoned the hospital about 5:00 p.m. and talked to my younger sister, Teedee, and she said that Eva did go to see the doctor and that he said Renee's lower bowels had collapsed but as soon as she started to have bowel movements again, she'll be O.K. and that there was no need for us to worry, because in a couple of days she'll be up and around. That was a big relief to me. The doctor said he knew that the family wanted to have her transferred to Vancouver, but he didn't think that was necessary. I told Teedee to come and get me with her car and bring me back to the hospital because I had supper ready to bring down to them.

Around 6:00 p.m. Renee had a bowel movement. I was very happy about this, and told her so. I said "Oh Boy Honey! You're going to start getting better." I went to get toilet paper but I couldn't find it so the nurse went and got one. Margaret returned to the room then and I told her that Renee just had a bowel movement and she was happy to hear that. Richard arrived to sit with Renee for the night and he hadn't eaten all day either. We said we would heat something up for him and Eva and I left.

About 10:00 p.m. I got a call to come to the hospital. I got dressed right away, phoned for a sitter for my little girl and ran all the way down to the hospital.

At 9:00 p.m. Richard had been sitting by his daughter's bedside. She told him the pains were getting worse and she seemed to be having trouble breathing. "Just take it easy, Babe," Richard said, stroking Renee's hair. "I'll get someone to come help you." He called a nurse and asked her to get the doctor. Dr. Pickup did not come to the hospital when he was telephoned but instead ordered two needles to be administered to the patient. One hour later Richard rang for the nurse, intending to ask again for the doctor as Renee's pains were getting worse. The nurse who answered his call looked at Renee, flung open the window and rushed out of the room. Dr. Pickup arrived a few minutes later and yelled for an oxygen tank. One was brought. It was empty. He yelled for another and began trying to listen to Renee's heart through his stethoscope. He flung the stethoscope down.

"It doesn't work. Get me another one!" he ordered.

The new oxygen tank arrived and the mask was placed over the little girl's face. By this time the rest of the family had arrived and they waited anxiously in the hallway as Richard and Margaret stood, terrified, by their daughter's bed.

Dr. Pickup turned to Richard. "It's too late. Her heart has stopped."

"Can't you get it going again?" Richard pleaded.

Dr. Pickup began heart massage, then poked at Renee's fingers a few times. "What are you doing, poking?" Richard sobbed contemptuously. "She's already dead."

The family, gathered at the bedside, broke down. Dr. Pickup ordered Nurse Heather George to get sedatives. When she returned with envelopes containing the usual three Seconal tablets per person, the doctor hollered at her: "That's not enough! Give them plenty! Make sure everybody has lots!"

After the shocked and grief-stricken family left the hospital, Nurse George found Dr. Pickup sitting in the patients' lounge. "He was crying," she said. "I didn't know what to say to him. He was under the influence of alcohol. He wasn't intoxicated. He said he would not sleep that night."

Two days later, on the evening of Wednesday, January 24th, mortician Leo O'Connell, from the nearby town of Campbell River, arrived in Alert Bay to prepare Renee's body for burial. Somewhat disturbed that her death certificate did not list a cause of death, he began the embalming process nonetheless. However, when he noticed scar tissue around the girl's vagina he became suspicious that she may have been sexually assaulted and, unsure of his legal responsibilities in such a situation, he stopped what he was doing and decided to think about it over dinner. After dinner, still uncertain and apprehensive, he drove around for a while. He stopped in at the hospital and asked one of the nurses if she knew anything about the Renee Smith death.

"The nurse told me that they thought the same as I did when the girl was a patient there...that she had been sexually assaulted. They said when they would go to visit the girl in her room to cover her up with a blanket or touch her, the girl would call out [a man's name and the words] 'Don't touch me any more...leave me alone.' ''

O'Connell decided to walk next door to the doctor's house to ask him about Renee's case. "When I got there the doctor was pretty well inebriated," O'Connell said later. "In fact, he was staggering around."

Dr. Pickup told him that no cause was listed on the death certificate because he still did not know why Renee had died and still hadn't decided what he was going to write on the death certificate. He told O'Connell that he had not notified the coroner and was not asking for an autopsy because, in his experience, he had found that Indians in general did not like autopsies and he felt that Renee's family, in particular, did not want an autopsy in this case. At O'Connell's insistence, Dr. Pickup agreed to accompany the mortician to the morgue to examine Renee's body.

"We both examined the girl's vagina. When Dr. Pickup looked at her, he said, 'Oh my God! I agree with you. I agree with you but I won't back you up. We both better go and talk about it at my house.' ''

Back at Pickup's home, the doctor tried to persuade the mortician to keep his suspicions to himself and to proceed with preparing Renee's body for burial.

"You'd just be opening a can of worms," Pickup told O'Connell. "Things like this happen all the time in Alert Bay and it's better to leave things alone."

Mrs. Pickup also tried to persuade O'Connell to proceed with embalming Renee's body. "She asked me what I thought I could prove anyway," O'Connell explained later.

"I don't care," O'Connell said he told the Pickups. "If you don't call the police, I will. I won't sleep to-night if I don't."

"I haven't slept since she died," Dr. Pickup mumbled in response.

O'Connell contacted the R.C.M.P. Staff Sergeant in charge of the Alert Bay Detachment, and the hospital administrator. The Sergeant, accompanied by a Constable, and the administrator joined the mortician and the doctor at the morgue. It was agreed that there appeared to be evidence of sexual assault and that therefore an autopsy should be conducted.

Ethel:

Thursday, January 25, 1979

I telephoned my sister Vera to get her out of bed at 8:15 this morning and she told me that the RCMP had confiscated the body, and that it was illegal to bury a person without the proper diagnosis of their death and that they said there had to be an autopsy. I was very upset and I went to Mum's. She told me that they were sending Renee's body away on the evening flight because they couldn't get her on the morning flight. She then told us to go and check on Margaret. We got up to Margaret's place and she and her husband were upset. She told us that the RCMP got them out of bed at 1:30 a.m. to question them further on the cause of Renee's death. Sergeant Barrie told them that the doctor had just reported her death to them at 11:30 that night and that she was sexually molested. The RCMP then went and got Richard's brother, Leonard, out of bed and brought him down to the police station until 5:30 a.m. getting a statement from him. He felt bad enough about Renee's death because he felt responsible for her. He was the one to babysit Margaret and Richard's children while we were in Reno.

What I couldn't understand was why the Doctor waited two days after her death to report it. It was so cruel of him. It was hard enough on the family having to lose Renee. Then to have something like this slapped on our faces. We put our trust on the Doctor, believing him when he told us there was nothing to worry about.

The autopsy established that death had been caused by severe generalized peritonitis resulting from a ruptured appendix.

"I made a very thorough examination and found no evidence of any problem with her sexual organs," the Vancouver pathologist who performed the autopsy stated. "There was no bruising in the vaginal area. I looked for scarring. There could have been scarring there but if there was it was very, very hard to assess and the healing had been excellent. I found no evidence whatsoever of sexual assault."

William Deadman, formerly a local magistrate and administrator of St. George's, and, in 1979, a trustee of the St. George's Hospital Society, husband of the hospital's medical records librarian, close friend and associate of Dr. Pickup's, and local coroner, received the results of the autopsy. He concluded that death was neither unnatural nor accidental, nor, in his opinion, had Renee's death been sudden or unexpected. Under the circumstances, he could see no reason to call an inquest.

NOTES:

Sources for this chapter are tape recordings, an account written by Ethel Scow, newspaper reports, personal notes, and Gottschau, Walter (ed) (1979), Transcript: *Inquest into the Death of Renee Bernice Smith held at the Alert Bay Coroner's Court*, April-June 1979, Vols. I & II.

CHAPTER 2

Action and Reaction

Cultural attitudes to violence differ—Indians do expect to suffer more pain, discomforts, disabilities and deformities because they fight more. There are more accidents and deaths. Infant mortality is high, but the loss of a child in an Indian community is accepted in an entirely different frame of mind than in a white man's society...
—The Canadian Health Care System: Students' and Teachers' Manual, Vol. 5, Canadian Hospitals Association, 1984, p. 50

Alert Bay, B.C.
February, 1979

No one in this Native community exists as an isolated individual. Everyone is someone else's mother, father, brother, sister, son, daughter, husband, wife, aunt, uncle, cousin, grandmother, grandfather, in-law. Experiences, no matter how personal in nature, are a property of the collectivity. No one remains untouched by either good times or bad times. The winter of 1978 had been a particularly bad time, remembered by most as a series of funerals.

There are social scientists who put forward the theory that groups of people who experience high mortality rates become somewhat desensitized to death. This has not been my experience. Each death in this community is more like fresh salt in wounds that never get a chance to heal.

35

Official causes of death among Alert Bay Natives during the 1970s conformed to the norm for Native communities across Canada. Alcohol-related accidents and violence took the lives of almost twice the percentage of young people as in the non-Native population; alcohol-related diseases accounted for the majority of the disproportionate number of deaths among the middle-aged, and, consequently, significantly fewer Native people reach old age than do non-Natives. Infant mortality, while declining, remained higher among Natives than among non-Natives.

There was growing evidence, however, in the experience of many of Dr. Pickup's patients, that the doctor's own drinking habit was cause for concern.

Dr. Pickup had the reputation of an "old country doctor" with a fondness for the bottle, and local people liked to tell stories—some amusing and some tragic—about errors made by Dr. Pickup when he treated patients while under the influence. The doctor himself made no secret of his drinking. My first job in "the Bay" was as a bar waitress, and the doctor was a familiar customer. A few years later, employed as a taxi driver, I often heard emergency calls from the hospital to "pick up Pickup at the Legion." A crusty, gruff man in his sixties, Dr. Pickup had a bedside manner that was blunt, brash, off-handed and, in the opinion of some Natives, offensive and racist. Complaints such as this one sent to the B.C. College of Physicians and Surgeons were typical:

On Monday, January 8, 1979, I went to a movie with my sister. Around 9:00 p.m. B.G. collapsed on his chair, and was immediately carried down to the lobby by his father and a friend. He was having a seizure. One of the workers called for an ambulance.

B. was brought to the hospital, and one of the Nurse's called for our only doctor. When he arrived, you could tell at first glance that he was under the influence of alcohol. He had to hang on to the wall, while he was walking towards us. The smell of alcohol was quite evident as he got closer. He tried to examine B. in his drunken stupor, but was almost unable to.

The Doctor started to complain to the father, H.G., that 97% of his Ambulance cases that he gets called in for never stay in the hospital for any more than 10 minutes. H.G. then said that this was the first time that B. has ever been an Ambulance case. Doctor Pickup then said that he was getting quite tired of us Indians, and called H. "Your nothing but a Goddamn Bastard." By this time we were all upset and just all walked out of there with B.

This was the first time that B.'s parents has ever experienced him having a seizure, and didn't know how to deal with the situation.

Maybe it was just a minor case with this certain patient. What would happen if there ever was such an emergency and the patient needed the doctor's care immediately. And he's just DRUNK.

As you are probably aware of, that Alert Bay is a small Community with a population of 1,500. And the Indians total more than half of that.

This is only one of the numerous incidents concerning our Indian people, and the Doctor.

Is there anyway that we could have him replaced? or to even have another Doctor here. We would feel so much safer.[1]

In 1976, three years before Renee died, one of her aunts, Louisa James,[2] entered St. George's for a hysterectomy and subsequently died from peritonitis following the operation. Mrs. James had been under Dr. Pickup's care, but a second doctor was also working out of the clinic at the time. A Native woman who was working at the hospital swore the following affidavit as to what took place.

I, E.M.E., Registered Nurse, of BELLA COOLA in the Province of British Columbia do solemnly declare I graduated as a nurse in 1973. I worked at Alert Bay Hospital for 6 months starting in January 1976.

Dr. Pickup had been out drinking at the Legion every night for some time. On the day of Louisa's operation, she was having a hysterectomy, Dr. Pickup was quite shakey. During the operation one of the other nurses opened the door to the O.R. and she said "E., I don't like what I heard in there." I asked her what happened but she wouldn't tell me. Three days post-op Louisa developed fever and pains all over her body. I suspected she was developing post-op complications. Some of the other nurses said she had a low pain tolerance. I never believed it. I had worked with her a lot.

A week later the Doctor ordered sutures to be removed. It was my duty to do that and I removed two sutures. The wound was gaping and draining foul smelling purulent discharge. Dr. Pickup saw the wound and said that it was good for it to drain.

Two days later, Dr. Pickup was leaving for Cokis Island on one of his regular visits. He had ordered 3 cc of Penicillin IM to be given to Louisa each a.m. I asked the nurse in charge to phone the other Doctor about Louisa. She refused because of Hospital policy. I waited until I was sure that Dr. Pickup had left the Hospital before I called the other Doctor. He came at once and examined the patient. He ordered I/V with antibiotic to be set up. He didn't say anything to me.

The next morning I reported what I had done to the Head Nurse. She said that I shouldn't have done it, and that I would get into trouble. About lunch time she came back and told me I had nothing to worry about. Louisa had a nicked bowel and had developed peritonitis. I was

37

coordinating an All Native Conference and I had to leave for Prince Rupert for 4 days. Louisa said "Hurry back."

On my way to the airport in Prince Rupert when I was leaving I met W.G. who was returning from Vancouver and I told her about it. I asked her to try and get Louisa to Vancouver. I also tried to get the Director of Nursing to persuade Dr. Pickup to transfer Louisa to Vancouver, but Dr. Pickup was stubborn.

When I returned from Prince Rupert I went straight to the hospital to see Louisa. She was having blood transfusions on both arms and legs. They tried to pump 21 pints of blood into her. The infection was so severe that it had burst the arteries and she was bleeding internally. Louisa died in hospital at Alert Bay about 13 days post-op.

At present I am bed ridden in Bella Coola Hospital but I am starting to sit up a bit. I would be willing to speak to an investigator if he or she comes to Bella Coola.

AND I make this solemn Declaration conscientiously believing it to be true, and knowing that it is of the same force and effect as if made under oath, and by virtue of the Canada Evidence Act.[3]

Many people in the Native community responded angrily to Louisa James' death, but Coroner Deadman requested neither an autopsy nor an inquest and Louisa's grieving husband asked that no further action be taken so that he and his six children could get on with rebuilding their lives. Those who had wanted to pursue the issue respectfully bowed to his wishes and the anger over Louisa's death became one more coal in the fire. Local representatives of the Indian Health Division of National Health and Welfare Canada assured the Nimpkish Band Council that the appropriate authorities had been notified of the circumstances surrounding Louisa's death, but the Band Council was never told about any action which may or may not have been taken.

During the Fall of 1978, a number of relatively minor incidents had taken place and Dr. Pickup seemed, publicly, to be drinking more heavily than usual. In December of 1978, the Hospital Board wrote to Dr. Pickup warning him that if a doctor was found treating patients while under the influence of alcohol his hospital privileges would be suspended. In that same month, the Kwakiutl District Council, representing all the Kwakwaka'wakw bands, with a total population of 3500 people, passed a resolution asking the B.C. College of Physicians and Surgeons to investigate Dr. Pickup. Renee's death the following month therefore caused a good deal of anger, as well as grief, within the Native community. For many, it was the last straw.

A small local radio station had been set up in Alert Bay in 1977 as part of the Canadian Broadcasting Corporation's commitment to service outlying communities and to develop Native programming and broadcasting facilities. Mark, an expatriate Californian who had been living in the area for several years and had had some experience in media, had been hired as researcher, reporter, broadcaster, and manager of the tiny one-room station which bumped the regular CBC service from 5:00 to 6:00 p.m. daily. As rumours flew around town about what had happened to Renee, Mark began trying to investigate.

One member of the St. George's Hospital Society Board of Trustees confided in Mark that the Board had discussed the Renee Smith "incident." She told him that "they [the Indians] should have gotten Dr. Pickup on the Louisa James case. They'll never get him on this one." And, despite having already received the results of the autopsy, she referred to the allegation of sexual assault as an issue which complicated discussions of the death. She refused to make any public statements.

Mark's discussions with other members of the Hospital Board were less informative. Most refused to speak to him at all. Coroner Deadman continued to insist that there had been nothing unusual about Renee's death and that therefore there was no need for an inquest. Representatives of the Vancouver Coroner's office, the College of Physicians and Surgeons, and federal and provincial ministries of health, passed the bureaucratic buck back and forth among themselves.

Mark came to see me about the investigations he had been making and we talked about what could be done. I had lived on the reserve for about six years, had worked for the Band Council and had been involved in various community organizing activities. I discussed with the Band Manager and a few of the Band Councillors the possibility of taking some action. Everyone agreed that something had to be done, once and for all, but the Councillors were uncomfortable about taking any public action not requested by Renee's family. In a situation as tragic as this, no one wanted to appear to be exploiting the family's grief for what could be seen as political purposes. They decided that anyone who wished, as a private individual, to pursue the issue, should go ahead. While the Band Council would support the action, it would not officially initiate it.

I got in touch with a band member, Renee Taylor, who was attending law school at the University of British Columbia. Renee, in turn, spoke privately with the band's legal advisor, Michael Jackson, who suggested that the first step would be to request that the Chief Coroner of B.C. override the local coroner's decision and order an inquest.

On February 9, 1979, two petitions were drawn up by a few people who could be described as community activists, including myself. One petition was addressed to the Attorney-General of B.C. and the other to the Minister of Health of B.C. We called ourselves the Concerned Citizens Group, to reflect the fact that non-Natives were among the initiators of the petitions (although all were allied in one way or another to the Native community) and to encourage as many people as possible to sign. Dr. Pickup and many of the St. George's Hospital Society and Board of Trustees were members of the old and entrenched colonial "white elite" whose local power base was substantial, and to whom many people in both communities, Native and non-Native, continued to show deference. Those of us who initiated the petitions quite specifically wished to avoid the inevitable polarization which we knew would take place if the issue was identified as an Indian/White political battle. Our objectives were pragmatic, and there was greater hope of success, we felt, if the problem was clearly defined as one of quality of medical care for all patients. The petitions read as follows:

To the Attorney-General of B.C.:
The recent death of a young female member of the Nimpkish Indian Band has resulted in considerable controversy in our community. This controversy has further eroded the confidence many people hold in the level of health care here.
We, the undersigned, feel strongly that an inquest into the death of Renee Smith is necessary to determine the cause of her death and to restore confidence in the health care system of our province.

To the Minister of Health of B.C.:
The tragic death here, during the very first weeks of the International Year of the Child, of an eleven-year-old female member of the Nimpkish Indian Band, has shocked our community.
The shock is the latest in a series of incidents which have seriously impaired the confidence of many residents in the quality of health care received here.
In order to identify the causes of this serious impairment of confidence, we beg you to undertake a full-scale inquiry into the delivery of medical services here in Alert Bay. In order to be effective this investigation would have to take into account our relative isolation and our particular historical and cultural situation.
We hope you and your department will choose a realistic and humane approach to this plea.
We trust we will hear from you soon.

Mark took the petitions to friends of his in the local and neighbouring White communities who he thought would be sympathetic, and I and a few others began to circulate them within the Native community. On February 10th, Renee's aunts (Margaret's sisters) started taking the petitions door-to-door on the reserve and by February 15th, 250 signatures had been collected, representing approximately 80 per cent of the adult residents of the reserve and several non-Natives as well. With a few notable exceptions such as the high school principal and a former Federal Indian Health Nurse, the 12 non-Native signatures from Alert Bay were those of recent arrivals, and employees of the Band and District

Councils. A few people from the neighbouring town of Sointula, also served by St. George's, signed as well.

Once Renee's family had endorsed the petitions the Nimpkish Band Council offered their official support and wrote to the College of Physicians and Surgeons of B.C., on February 14, 1979, as follows:

Sirs:

As representatives of the Indian people residing at Alert Bay, we would like to express our concern regarding medical care available on this island. Specifically the quality of care as delivered by Dr. Pickup. It has been apparent for some time that the Doctor has a drinking problem.

As a group attempting to deal with the many social problems on our reserve, we are well aware of the effect that alcoholism has on a persons ability to function or perform their work effectively.

Because of our location and the financial situation of most Indian families, any Doctor working here literally has a captive clientele. We would like to assure our people that the care they are receiving is not sub-standard but are not able to do this at this time.

The death of an Indian child from a ruptured appendics last month has resulted in a petition from many residents of the Island to have Dr. Pickup removed. Many racist remarks attributed to Dr. Pickup at that time have also shocked and horrified us.

We request that your organization assist us in our efforts to ensure that adequate health care is available to the people of this reserve.[4]

Other people with complaints, Native and non-Native, were encouraged to write individually to the College, and many did. Those who felt confident about doing so, wrote letters about experiences they had had with Dr. Pickup and St. George's, while some dictated their stories and signed their names to the typed transcripts that others prepared.

Signed transcript:

R: How long have you lived in Alert Bay?
J: I've got to think...15 years I've been living in Alert Bay but even before that when I was in my home town village I used to come over here to see Dr. Pickup so I've been going to him all my life.
R: When was the first time you went to him about your eye trouble?
J: When it first got itchy and it was all red and I got worried about it right away because I never had eye trouble before. He gave me eye drops and the funny part about it was how he tested my eyes.
R: What did he do?

41

J: He just put his finger like that and pulled my eye lid down and he told me it was an allergy of some kind.

R: Did he say what kind?

J: No, he didn't know what was wrong. I kept on asking him everytime I went to see him.

R: So that was when it first started...then you got the drops?

J: Yes and I used them everyday. 3 times a day—that's what he told me to do. I did that for about 5 days and then after the week-end was over I went to see him on a Monday. That was the second time I went. That time he told me to keep on using the same eye drops.

R: When you went back to him that Monday, the second time, were your eyes still the same? Was it worse or better?

J: It was really itchy and it really bothered me and I kept on rubbing them and it was all red—the bottom part was all red...

R: So when you went back to him the second time did he examine your eyes the second time?

J: He did the same as the first time. He just pulled my lower lid down and looked at it. And he told me that same thing...that it was an allergy of some kind and to keep taking the same drops.

R: What happened then? Did you keep taking the drops?

J: Yes I did but I kind of slowed down on them because I was scared to use them because it wasn't helping. It didn't stop the itching and the redness didn't go away.

R: How long did that go on then?

J: For five weeks altogether.

R: How long did you keep going to Pickup?

J: I went to him once a week for all five weeks. The third time I went was when he changed my eyedrops and that's when my vision started to go. It was after that third time.

R: When your vision started to go blurry did he ever examine you any more than just pulling your lid down?

J: Yes, he did. He used a flashlight. You know those penlights. That's all he used and then he told me to keep on using the drops and I told him about my headaches too because they were getting worse and he just gave me 292s.

R: So then what did you do?

J: Dr. Pickup told me to go see a specialist in Comox and H. took me down right away. But it was already too late. But he managed to save some of my sight.

R: What did the doctor in Comox say when you saw him?

J: I should ask H. about that name...the eye disease I have...There are three different names for it...I remember something like 'itis' and something about 'retina' but the doctor in Comox said that if I had got the right treatment or if he sent me down that first week I would have been all right to-day.

R: What treatment did you receive in Comox?

J: He gave me 24 pills to take that night that I got down there and about 6 different kinds of eyedrops-every five minutes all night that first night I was there and it improved my eyesight right away but that's as far as it went. I was in hospital for 2 months in St. Joseph's in Comox. They were treating me. I had an injection—cortisone which helped clear up the infection because it got really bad in both eyes—behind my eyes. It got really bad and it damaged the tissue behind my eyes...

Sometimes it makes me so mad when I think that I could have been all right to-day if he had sent me down right away. I'm not the type to go to the Doctor every week and he knows that. He knows me. He should have known it was serious when I kept coming back. I was really worried about my eyes. Thats why I kept on going.

R: What percentage of your eyesight do you have left?

J: I forget what they told me. But everything is just blurry and I can't see anything clearly at all.

R: Did you ever go back to Dr. Pickup after this?

J: No, I haven't. I've never gone back. I won't go back to him for anything. Even if I get sick I won't go. Sometimes I just sit here and cry when I want to do things that I can't do anymore...It's all on account of his—oh, I don't know. You know, just the way he is, that's all. I finally had seven specialists looking at me in Vancouver and they were just shaking their heads about how Pickup could have let it go that long. They said he should have sent me down right away...

I used to really love to embroider and now I can't do that at all anymore.[5]

Sirs:

I would like to express my deep concerns about the medical care that is received in Alert Bay at St. George's Hospital.

I worked in the hospital as a registered nurse for five months from March 31st to August 31st, 1977. There exists no doubt in my mind that Dr. H. J. Pickup is an alcoholic. When I worked nights and evenings there was not one time when he came in sober. No one under the influence of alcohol is capable of giving optimum care to human beings.

My concern is for the people of Alert Bay who are unable to go elsewhere for care. This is the trend for those who can afford it. My concern is also for people who have medical and surgical emergencies. There is only one doctor on this island and we are cared for by him under the influence of his illness, his alcoholism.[6]

Signed transcript:

My son was to have his tonsils removed when he was four years old, so I brought him in to the Hospital, St. George's Hospital. On the day that he was operated on he didn't come out of anesthesia in the afternoon and that made me very anxious and worried for him. He looked so pale and withdrawn. I stayed all day and then went home for supper, I had this nagging feeling that wouldn't set me at ease, because I kept thinking of my baby. So I returned to the hospital at 7:00 p.m. visiting hours.

When I got there my baby still had not woken up and there was blood showing at the corner of his mouth, and he was paler and then I panicked. I asked if he had woken up yet, and the answer was no, I asked where the Doctor was and why my baby hadn't come out of anesthesia beause it had been too long. Dr. Pickup arrived and told me that there was nothing to worry about. I didn't believe him and I started to cry and scream at him to check S. over because I saw that he was bleeding, and he argued that he would be alright. But when he checked him, I knew something had gone wrong when the nurses were running around. They had to do a transfusion. I was so terrified at this time that there was nothing to do but pray. My son made it through this crisis, and the next day the head nurse in charge commended me about my action. She also told me that if I hadn't insisted that he be checked he would have died, because he had lost so much blood.

So after these experiences I was always afraid. It was only after fighting for my rights that whenever I myself landed in the hospital The Doctor would give me a special nurse.[7]

To Whom it may Concern,

In regards to the level of adequate Medical Care being provided by Dr. Pickup, I will relate the following two incidents:

1) Between 1965-1966 I was being treated by Dr. Pickup, at St. George's for pain I was experiencing under my Rib cage, on both sides. During this time I was put into hospital 3 times (about one month each time) and was being treated for a gaseous stomach. After the third time in the hospital, Dr. Pickup told me not to come back, as it was just a gaseous stomach.

The pain continued, so I went to Vancouver, and saw a Doctor suggested by my father. He examined me and diagnosed gall-stones. As soon as a hospital bed was open, he operated and removed them.

2) In the early fall of 1978 my daughter aged 10 years old was molested in the early hours of the morning. The following afternoon

44

I brought her to the hospital and tried to get her in to see the Doctor. The Nurse in charge asked me the reason, and I spoke quietly, as the Waiting Room was crowded, and told her someone had tried to fool around with my daughter. She rudely asked me to repeat it in a louder voice. I started to speak, and then she cut me off, and told me to bring her on the following Monday. I returned on Monday, and saw the Doctor (Which was Dr. Pickup). He said he wasn't going to examine her as it was too long after the incident to prove anything, and besides my daughter was already upset enough.

If a situation arose where I had to see a Doctor in Alert Bay, and another one was available, I would rather not see Dr. Pickup.[8]

Dear Sirs:

The following incident happened to me during my sixth month of pregnancy. I suspected I might have a bladder infection, so I made an appointment with Dr. Jack Pickup at which time Mrs. Pickup asked why I wanted to see him and I told her of suspected bladder infection. When I saw Dr. Pickup, he said "Why do you think you might have bladder infection?" I said "Because I have had it before and I feel some familiar symptoms." He began to write out a prescription. I asked what the prescription was for and he replied that it was for a sulfa drug. So I said "I had trouble with kidney infection about ten years ago and I remember problems with sulfa drugs then." Dr. Pickup proceeded to tear up the prescription and write another one for a penicyllin drug. This prescription was given to me without having done any examination or urinalysis.

I relate these events to illustrate my lack of confidence in Dr. Pickup and dread that I should have to rely on his competency in an emergency situation. You can verify these details by writing or calling my regular doctor in Vancouver, Dr. _____ at this address and phone number.[9]

Sirs:

I am in full support of the inquest concerning the death of Renee Smith. I have for years questioned the abilities and ethics of Dr. Pick-up who was the doctor involved in her death.

About six years ago I was employed by the Band Council...[of one of the outlying villages]...as a welfare aide and was quite involved in the medical, economic and social aspect of the people in...[that]...village.

At the insistance of a community member, I was asked to meet with Dr. Pick-up and herself as she felt quite intimidated by him. She wanted to know what his diagnoses of her illness was as she had not been told.

So I met with her and Dr. Pick-up. He proceeded to talk about her person in a very derogatory way and he did not appear to care that she was sitting in the same room. It was as if she were not even present. I, in turn, lost my temper and reminded him that he was acting in a very unprofessional manner and that he had no right making value judgements on patients, especially when he was not aware of her economic and living conditions.

As a result of these problems with Dr. Pick-up and from what other people have told me I have made it a point to stay away from him for any medical care. When I am ill I try to cure myself or leave town to get medical attention.

Thank you for your attention on this matter.[10]

To Whom It May Concern:

Re: Dr. Pickup

Five years ago, when my youngest daughter was four years old, she fell on her chest just before supper. Later in the evening, about 10:30 p.m., she woke up crying with pains in her chest. I brought her to the emergency ward at the hospital. The nurses called the doctor on call, Dr. Pickup. He came over after fifteen minutes of complaining about being called at such a late time and without examining her, told me that there was nothing to be done until morning and I could leave her in the hospital, in fact I should leave her there....

Another incident: my youngest child suddenly broke out in an extreme case of hives all over his body about 9:30 one evening. Because we could not alleviate his itching and discomfort, I brought him into the hospital. Dr. Pickup came in obviously enebriated. The other doctor came in right after and talked Dr. Pickup out of the nursing station and took over.

Another incident: When I was in the maternity ward almost five years ago Dr. Pickup came into the ward one morning about 12:30-1:00 a.m.—very enebriated—"to make his rounds". I was not in his care at the time but there were four other women in the ward. One of the nurses came in to usher him out.

I find it an intolerable situation when I have three children whose health care is almost nil because I do not trust the local doctor. Right now I have a young son whose throat is swollen and because I work I must wait or find the most convenient time to go to Port McNeil or Port Hardy. With these two factors constantly hanging over my head I feel that *someone* should do *something* to insure safety and security of healthcare of every resident here in Alert Bay.[11]

Dear Sirs/Madams,

I'm writing this letter to protest the quality of health care that our native peoples are receiving from the local doctor in Alert Bay. I speak of Dr. Pickup.

I have seen Dr. Pickup drunk quite often during the hours of 8:00 A.M. to 4:30 P.M. I have also seen him quite often drunk in the evenings. Common sense tells me that this man has a drinking problem.

What evidence do I have to substantiate this you ask? The evidence I have is my talking to our people about their wounds. They have told me that this doctor has treated them while drunk and often done a poor job as a result. I believe them.

When I see this man always drinking it leads me to believe that he is deteriating as a man. Which also means as a doctor. I have seen other men crumble the same way. I've seen how drinking affects their work. I can hardly believe that doctors are exempt.

The people I speak for...want you to take my words for what they are. If...their words you don't trust, as mine you don't trust...my letter to you then will have been a waste of time.[12]

In mid-March our petitions to the Attorney-General and the Minister of Health were acknowledged as follows:

Ladies and Gentlemen:

I wish to acknowledge the receipt of your letter and expression of concern containing the signatures of a considerable number of residents in the Alert Bay area.

Concerning the tragic death of Miss Renee Smith, I have been informed that Coroner Deadman has ordered a complete investigation into the matter, and an autopsy has been held.

Also the Supervising Coroner for the Province of British Columbia, Mr. Glen McDonald, will preside at a public inquest which is tentatively set for April 18, 1979, at Alert Bay.

Thank you for drawing this matter to my attention, and may I please express my sympathy to all members of your community, and family and friends of Miss Smith.

Yours very truly,

Garde B. Gardom

Attorney-General of B.C.

To Concerned Citizens of Alert Bay:

I have your petition of February 9, 1979, expressing concerns for health services in Alert Bay. I am informed that the matter has been formally brought to the attention of the College of Physicians and Surgeons and that Dr. J. A. Hutchison, Registrar, will be conducting an enquiry and will be visiting Alert Bay....I am also informed that the Supervising Coroner...will be ordering an inquest.

Both these processes are in accord with the responsibilities and jurisdictions of the two offices already involved. Neither the Attorney-General nor myself need therefore to override the Coroner and the College of Physicians and Surgeons. We are, however, concerned about the issues you raised and wish to assure you of our continuing interest in ensuring a satisfactory solution.

Dr. K. I. G. Benson has been appointed Health Officer for the Upper Island Health Unit and has advised me that he will be in the Unit area before the end of this month and has already scheduled a visit to Alert Bay....

Yours sincerely,

R. H. McClelland

Minister of Health for B.C.

In the meantime, the petitions and their implications had created quite a stir in Alert Bay and the surrounding communities.

St. George's Hospital served the outlying Native villages in the Kwakwaka'wakw area, the neighbouring non-Native communities of Sointula and Port McNeill, and the surrounding logging camps as well as Alert Bay itself. There was a clinic in Port McNeill, on Vancouver Island, with a full-time doctor in attendance who had hospital privileges at St. George's, and Dr. and Mrs. Pickup travelled to Sointula, located on adjacent Malcolm Island, on Wednesdays, to see patients there. Both Port McNeill and Sointula are approximately forty minutes travelling time from Alert Bay, on the same ferry run. Emergency cases were brought by ferry or air ambulance to St. George's in Alert Bay, or, in more serious cases, were flown to hospitals in Campbell River, Victoria or Vancouver.

Dr. Pickup, while serving as Medical Director of St. George's, leased his own private clinic next door to the hospital, with office space and examining facilities for two doctors. Dr. Pickup had had several long-term partners since he began practising in Alert Bay in 1949, but during the past decade there had been a parade of "second doctors" through the clinic, few of whom had lasted more than a year. Second doctors usually found that they were only given the overflow appointments and therefore could not make enough money to make their practice worthwhile. Young doctors complained that since most serious problems were treated by doctors and hospitals off the island, they did not have an opportunity to treat a wide enough range of maladies to sufficiently develop their skills. In January of 1979, when Renee Smith died, Dr. Pickup had been the sole medical practitioner on the island for eighteen months, during which time he had been on call twenty-four hours a day, seven days a week.

A small circle of Dr. Pickup's closest friends and associates rallied to his defence immediately, and, apparently subscribing to the theory that "the best defence is a good offence," did so by attacking the personal character of the people who initiated the petitions, and by expressing derogatory opinions about the Indian community in general. Others in the White community opted to take a more "neutral" stance, acknowledging that there was a problem but torn either by personal loyalty to Dr. Pickup, or to their end of town, or both. Some privately supported the petitions but assured themselves that going public wasn't really necessary as now that an inquest had been called, they were confident that the truth would come out and the matter would be dealt with by the proper authorities. A very few openly supported the petition campaign.

There were Native people, too, who were initially reluctant to become involved in any action against Dr. Pickup. But what haunted these people was the knowledge that Renee could have been their daughter. Most, therefore, knowing the risks they were taking, signed. Some, however, openly supported Dr. Pickup and refused to sign either of the petitions.

One Native woman, who worked at St. George's in the winter of 1979, told me later how she felt:

> Well when Kelly came to me with the petition, well, I sure didn't want to sign, you know. I just started work and I'd been gone from the Bay for a long time and I just thought I don't want no trouble, you know. Just stay on everyone's good side and stay out of fights. I figure that's how you get along in this town, hey? But, well, you kind of had to sign it, hey? I mean everyone knows it's all true and it was only right to sign, hey?

NOTES:

[1]Government of Canada, Department of National Health and Welfare, Medical Services/Indian Health Division, (1980) transcript of proceedings, *In the Matter of An Inquiry into Health and Health Care in Alert Bay, B.C.*, Dr. G. Goldthorpe, Commissioner, Vol. II, pp. 323-325. This source will be referenced from now on as "*The Goldthorpe Inquiry*," (1980) Transcript:...."

While this letter was read into the public record at *The Goldthorpe Inquiry*, the writer of this letter is still resident in Alert Bay where Dr. Pickup remains, often, the sole medical practitioner. In cases such as this one, where particular individuals were not key or leading participants, I have opted to identify people by initials only, or by pseudonym.

[2]Pseudonym. Again, this affidavit and the details of this incident are part of the public record. However, "Mrs. James'" family did not voluntarily place themselves in the public eye, and specifically chose not to take any action regarding this. In view of the sensitive nature of the case, and out of respect for their feelings, I use a pseudonym.

[3]*The Goldthorpe Inquiry*, (1980) Transcript: Vol. II, pp. 313-316.

[4]Nimpkish Band Council, Public Information Package, distributed August 12, 1979.

[5]*The Goldthorpe Inquiry*, (1980) Transcript: Vol. II, pp.362-374.

[6]Ibid., 377-378.

[7]Ibid., 409-411.

[8]Ibid., 432-434.

[9]Ibid., 359-360.

[10]Ibid., 379-381.

[11]Ibid., 449-451.

[12]Ibid., 339-341.

CHAPTER 3

My Country 'Tis of Thy People You're Dying

Alert Bay, B.C.
April, 1979

On April 7, 1979, the Kwakiutl District Council held a special meeting of representatives of all the Kwakwaka'wakw bands to discuss the recently announced cutbacks in federal funding to Indian health services. On the agenda of the All-Bands meeting was the Annual Report by the Public Health Nurse employed by the Indian Health Division of National Health and Welfare Canada.

This Federal Indian Health Nurse, Vera Robinson, had arrived in Alert Bay only a month before, in March, but quickly made herself known by her outspoken condemnation of Dr. Pickup and the hospital administration and nursing staff. She was equally critical of her own superiors and colleagues in the Medical Services/Indian Health Division of National Health and Welfare Canada for their collusion in the situation. Vera also frankly supported the band's initiatives in social and economic development, and education. Health Nurses were usually very reluctant to voice criticisms of either the medical establishment or their civil service employers, and customarily maintained a co-operative, but arm's length, relationship with the Band Council.

While previous Federal Indian Health Nurses had also been aware of the problems with Dr. Pickup and the hospital that were now being voiced, they had opted to deal with the situation by reporting to their own superiors, or by voicing their concerns to the doctor and the hospital administration privately, and/or by telling patients to put their complaints in writing to the College of Physicians and Surgeons, or to the Hospital's Board of Trustees. However, the College's method of handling such complaints was to forward a copy of the patient's letter to the physician in question, and since the Hospital Board was made up of local people known to be close to Dr. Pickup, with no encouragement other than this advice, few patients were prepared to take such an individual risk in a one-doctor town. Vera's unusually courageous position, therefore, earned her the immediate respect of the Indian community, particularly those members of the community who were involved in band administration, health and social services, and community development.

After submitting her report to the Kwakiutl District Council, Vera asked if she could present it to the public by means of the local radio station. Permission was granted.

Everyone in town listened to Haddington Reef Radio's one-hour show from 5:00 to 6:00 p.m. daily. The program announced upcoming events, interviewed local people, let the aspiring singers, songwriters and other performers of the area have a go at the microphone, invited school children on to sing and recite poems, and generally tried to please everyone most of the time.

To-day's program was different. At precisely 5:00 p.m. a voice announced solemnly: "This is Haddington Reef Radio." Pause. Then Buffy Sainte-Marie's husky voice blared bitterly out of radios in houses from one end of the island to the other, singing:

Now that your big eyes are finally opened
Now that you're wondering how must they feel
Meaning them that you've chased 'cross America's
movie screens!
Now that you're wondering how can it be real
that the ones you've called colourful, noble and proud
in your school propaganda
 they starve in their splendour
You've asked for my comment
I simply will render:
My country 'tis of thy people you're dying!

George, his cousin Kelly, and I were driving home after picking up our mail at the Post Office. We stared at each other, eyes wide, listening as the song went on, the intensity in Buffy Sainte-Marie's voice deepening as she spat out the words:

...You force us to send our toddlers away
to your schools where they're taught
to despise their traditions
Forbid them their languages
Then further say

52

That American history really began
When Columbus set sail out of Europe
And stress
that the nation of leeches that's conquered this land
are the biggest, and bravest and boldest and best.
And yet
Where in your history books is the tale
of genocide basic to this country's birth
of the preachers who lied
how the Bill of Rights failed...

"Oh no!" I groaned apprehensively, as visions raced through my mind of these words reverberating from Royal Family silver spoon collections and filling spotless arborite kitchens—on both ends of town.

Then came Vera's deep, flat, north-of-England voice:

I'm 'ere to read the report I delivered to-day to the Kwakiutl District Council. Many things should be said. There are many concerns. Maybe it is sufficient to quote the little child who spoke to Pearl and who simply asked: Why is it that only Indians die?

George pulled the car over to the side of the road and we sat frozen in our seats, ears glued to the radio.

Is that true? Is it only Indians who die? We found from our files that in two years, from January '77 to January '79, one white man died. He had cancer.

Forty-four Indians died.

The white man came from a population of approximately 600, the 44 Indians came from a population of approximately 1200. The child's statement is true. One white man in 600 means there should have been two Indian deaths. Why 44?

  1 did die from cancer
  8 did die of old age
  1 was a premature infant
  2 were small babies
  2 were young children
    one of which died of malnutrition
  1 died from a ruptured appendix, an eleven-year-old
  1 died of the effects of T.B.
  1 died of pneumonia
  1 from a blood condition
  1 from a brain infection

2 died from heart attacks
1 was a mental defective
1 died from a stroke

That is 22. What of the other 22?

4 between 23 and 46 drowned while under the influence of alcohol
3 aspirated while drunk
they were 26, 28, 34
5 between the ages of 57 and 69 died of liver failure due to alcohol
poisoning
2 were murdered while drunk—stabbed to death
3 young adults killed themselves while under the influence of alcohol

This is a report from a Health Office, not a death office, so we should report that in the same two years there were 55 births.

We do have the facts. Alcohol is the common factor that cannot be denied.

Do we have other health problems?

Yes we do. We had a large number of households that had at least one person sick with hepatitis. The hospital states that 90% of the in-patients were there because of alcohol abuse and now we are wondering why T.B. is on the increase and why people have high blood mercury levels.

This office, if it is to be a Health Office, needs some direction. We could give you more facts of people we know who will die shortly. We can be confident of their deaths. How can we be confident of your health?

1 in 600
44 in 1200

What is it going to be for January '79 to January '81?

That little child asked a question. We have to give the answer today even though it hurts. It is true, for Alert Bay, that only Indians die. Little child, how old will you be when you die? Please let us work together, to let you have the chance to live to a proud, happy, healthy old age.

We had heard this report at the District Council meeting and, depressing as it was, it differed little from the standard reports delivered by Public Health Nurses on a regular basis, which always concentrated on mortality statistics, alcohol abuse and child neglect. However, Vera went on to say that as a nurse responsible for Indian health she could no longer in all conscience refer Native patients to the local health personnel or facilities. When asked to explain her reasons for this rather drastic decision, she said:

> I am very much distressed with, like I say, the very low age at which people are dying. I am distressed with a few things I find in the hospital situation. I have written to the College of Physicians and Surgeons about that asking for an explanation because at the moment I cannot refer people there....I do not have the confidence that they will receive the care they need there...There are a lot of rumours but I am not interested in rumours. I have some facts of my own....I would like to challenge the Hospital Board....They are the people responsible for giving physicians their privileges....

Vera's broadcast implied that there was a direct link between the ratio of White to Indian deaths, and medical care at St. George's, and the erroneous impression given by her report was that Indians were being systematically slaughtered at St. George's. The Chief of the Nimpkish Band, Roy Cranmer, and Mayor Popovich of the Municipality, issued a joint press release in an attempt to correct this impression, but it was too late. Members of the Hospital Board rushed down to the radio station demanding time to rebut. They were given it, but it was too late. The Band Council demanded that Indian Health/Medical Services equip a clinic on the reserve and send a doctor up immediately to service the Indian community who, obviously, could not now be expected to continue to see Dr. Pickup. Medical Services complied, frightened that they too would be up for criticism, which they were.

I felt as though we had just watched someone plant a mine, and we were waiting for it to explode. Despite all the turmoil going on within the town, until Vera's broadcast the "Pickup business" had been presented to the "outside world" only in the official form of the petitions which had been sent to cabinet ministers, and personal letters or signed transcripts addressed to the College of Physicians and Surgeons. We were still shaky about the magnitude of what we had done and what it meant in a local context. Knowing the opposition we faced, we had tried up to this point to tread very delicately. Now, however, the media became involved and the battle became public. We had taken the plunge and there was no turning back.

Of course, upon scrutiny—and in hindsight—Vera's careless use of statistics and the exaggerated sensationalism of her presentation are obvious. Vera neglected to mention, for example, that of the 1200 Indians on the band lists, almost half did not live on reserves in Alert Bay, and many of the deaths she described did not take place in Alert Bay or at St. George's. Vera defended her position by arguing that there was, in fact, a clear connection between the mortality statistics and the quality of local medical care. She told reporters:

55

Good health care would challenge the drunkenness which contributes to tuberculosis and social ills in Alert Bay....This situation existed long before my arrival last month. I was the one who decided to take a stand....This community needs some help, it needs some direction.

It was true that in everyone's experience Indians certainly did do a lot more dying in Alert Bay than White people did, so to people unfamiliar with the ins and outs of "statistical tests of significance," and critical of medical care at St. George's, the point Vera was making made intuitive sense. It was a fact that alcohol abuse was, directly or indirectly, the major cause of death within the Native population, and it was also true, as Vera charged, that alcoholics admitted to the hospital were simply given a rest and some pills, and were then sent out for a few months until they inevitably returned to the hospital. From this point of view, Vera's argument—that the lack of serious attention the hospital gave to effectively treating what was ailing the vast majority of their patients contributed to the high mortality rates—seemed credible. Furthermore, Vera was, after all, a health care professional, and those of us who were involved in circulating the petitions were not, therefore we deferred to Vera's expertise in such matters. To an already simmering town, Vera's broadcast generated the extra heat needed to bring things to the boiling point.

The press—national T.V., radio and newspapers—flew in on chartered seaplanes and began questioning anyone they could find. Trying to be very cautious and painstakingly accurate, Pearl Alfred, the Band Manager, and I, told the press:

> The problem has been of concern to many villagers for some time and the time for action is long overdue....
>
> There is a considerable lack of confidence among citizens about the standard of health care available on the island....
>
> There is a lot of concern by both the Native and the non-Native population....
>
> This is not an attack on the hospital....
>
> The decision to seek a full-scale inquiry is not a personal smear campaign, but we have to face facts....
>
> We are sorry we had to go this route, but it's reached the point where we have to stand and make a decision....
>
> Many people regret having to seek the doctor's resignation but it has reached a point where we had to make a choice....

Rumours began to fly around town that all the doctors in the district were now going to refuse to work at St. George's since they felt that the petitions asking for an inquest and an inquiry had cast aspersions on their professional competence. Without any doctors, of course, the hospital would not be able to function and no one wanted to see the hospital closed down. Not only was St. George's a major employer of Native as well as non-Native people, but having a hospital in Alert Bay had always been important to the Native community because it allowed patients to remain close to home where they could be surrounded by supportive family and friends rather than being sent, isolated and alone, to relatively lonely city hospitals. Panic set in, on both ends of the island, at the prospect that the hospital would surely be closed down. Another petition was circulated in order to stop the rumours. This one read:

(1) We, the undersigned, consider Dr. Harold Pickup of Alert Bay, B.C. to be no longer capable of competently performing his duties as a general physician. We have chosen to take ourselves and our children to other doctors for medical care, at personal expense and inconvenience, rather than be treated by Dr. Pickup. We demand to have adequate medical care available in our community.

(2) A good deal of confusion has arisen out of the present controversy surrounding medical services in Alert Bay and at St. George's Hospital. We the undersigned wish to clarify the following points.

(a) our dissatisfaction is with the services provided in recent years by Dr. Pickup.

(b) we fully support the continuing operation of St. George's Hospital, on condition that medical personnel deserving of the community's trust, confidence and respect are secured.

(c) we are not calling into question the competence of any doctor having privileges at St. George's Hospital other than Dr. Harold Pickup.

(d) we demand the resignation of Dr. Harold Pickup on the basis that a large section of the community has lost confidence in his ability to practice medicine competently.

This lack of confidence has been growing over the past several years due primarily to Dr. Pickup repeatedly treating people while under the influence of alcohol and making racist comments to and about local Native people.

People who have either personally experienced such incidents or who have heard about them over and over again, naturally fear utilizing the hospital as long as Dr. Pickup is in charge.

Throughout the month of April 1979, the battle raged on. An ex-nurse, and now president of the Ladies' Auxiliary of St. George's Hospital, circulated a counter-petition which read:

We, the undersigned wish to make known that the care and attention given to us while in St. George's Hospital, here in Alert Bay, is of the finest in Canada and that we consider our community very fortunate to have Dr. H. J. Pickup as our physician and medical advisor.

Much ado was made of the fact that several Indians were among the approximately 200 signatories to this petition. Several of these people claimed, however, that they had signed because they had understood the petition to be in support of the continued operation of the hospital and not Dr. Pickup. This interpretation was supported by a woman from a neighbouring non-Native community who wrote to the Chairman of the Hospital Board and sent a copy of her letter to the Nimpkish Band Council and the Concerned Citizens Group:

> Dear Sir:
> ...I have questioned some of the people who signed the petition in support of Dr. Pickup here in Sointula, and the following was the result:
> (1) Yes, they agreed he had been a good doctor when he first practiced here.
> (2) Yes, they would go to him if they had a cold.
> (3) No, they would go to Vancouver if they felt they were really sick.
> (4) No, they did not think he was a competent doctor to-day.
> (5) Yes, it is common knowledge that Dr. Pickup is often under the influence of alcohol when he is treating patients.
> Surely the Board is not going to deny that they are aware of these facts and statements. Such a denial would be absolutely ludicrous.
> I do not question Dr. Pickup's competence from hearsay and gossip, but from personal experience.[1]

Most non-Natives who agreed with this woman, however, chose to remain silent, confiding in friends that they couldn't risk taking a public position.

Vera's report and radio broadcast proved to be a significant turning point in what was shaping up to be one of the biggest battles the town had ever seen. It also marked the point at which a crucial expansion took place in the very definition of the problem being addressed. While Vera accused the doctor and the hospital staff of general incompetence and unprofessionalism, and of economic self-interest in over-admitting Indian patients, hospitalizing them for unnecessarily long periods of time, and not effectively treating alcoholism, she also chastised them for allowing Indians to use the hospital in the ways some did. She believed that this perpetuated deficient life-styles and a lack of personal responsibility within the Native population. In other words, Vera felt that a major part of a health professional's obligations to patients was to change their life-styles. The issue now, therefore, came to include the question not only of the doctor's alcoholism but also that of the patients.

Up to this point the complaints, as they had been articulated in the petitions and in the letters and affidavits individuals had submitted, and as they had been formally and informally stated by Band representatives, had been:

(1) Dr. Pickup was responsible for Renee's death and should be held accountable for it. Of course, the circumstances of Louisa James' death in 1976 were still fresh in everyone's mind. Many felt that if they had taken a stand then, Renee might not have been lost.

(2) It had been common, public knowledge for a long time that Dr. Pickup was frequently under the influence of alcohol when he practised medicine, and that the time had come for this situation to be brought to an end.

(3) Many Natives, and some non-Natives, thought that the hospital's medical staff and Board of Trustees, as well as the various levels of government involved in funding medical services, had been ignoring, or covering up for, Dr. Pickup for years. Those of us who had circulated the petition asking for a public inquiry into the delivery of health care felt that they, and their employers, should be held accountable for the consequences of their conduct, and should not be allowed to continue these practices. In our view, since Indians formed the bulk of the patient population, it was they who were paying the price for problems in the system, while medical personnel enjoyed good salaries as well as social prestige, despite the fact that they were not living up to their own official standards. Many of us felt that the reason such a situation had been allowed to develop, and to continue, was because most of the patients were, in the eyes of those we held responsible, "only Indians anyway."

(4) Some people, mainly those working in health care and social services, complained about the revolving-door type of treatment alcoholics were receiving, the disproportionate length of time Indians were kept in hospital for relatively minor ailments, and the free-wheeling manner with which drugs were prescribed and dispensed. Again, the perpetuation of these practices was seen as serving the interests of the hospital and its staff whom we saw as the beneficiaries of the system. We didn't see the chronic alcoholics who were patients deriving any benefits from the situation, since they weren't getting any healthier and certainly didn't lead lives anyone would envy.

When the problem had been primarily defined as one of Dr. Pickup's drinking while on call and on duty, and his open contempt for many Indian patients, everyone, including his most dedicated supporters, had no choice but to be a bit sheepish. These charges were, as no one could deny, public knowledge. The explicit characterization of the issue as being an Indians vs. Whites conflict, however, and the expansion of the definition of the problem to include Indian alcoholism and health in general, had several major consequences.

First of all, some non-Natives, and not a few Natives, who had been reluctant to support the petitions but who had been unable, in good conscience, to refuse, now said that while they had supported the call for an inquest and an inquiry, and had agreed that something should be done about Dr. Pickup's drinking and about the hospital staff's lax attitude towards procedural rules and regulations, supporting accusations of the magnitude alluded to in Vera's broadcast was further than they were willing to go. Nor were they prepared to lend their support, they said, if it was going to be "turned into" a racial issue. It was a bit far-fetched, they argued, to blame the doctor and the hospital staff for alcoholism among Indians.

No one in the Indian community questioned the fact that excessive use of alcohol was the main immediate cause of most illness and death on the reserve. How could they? It was, after all, the people on the reserve who lived with these problems on a daily basis. Ever since alcohol had first been introduced during eighteenth-and nineteenth-century fur trade, there had been people and organizations among coastal Indians who tried in various ways to control and limit its abuse. Such efforts were, naturally, still being carried on formally and informally in 1979. The complaint regarding alcohol treatment at St. George's was, initially, simply that the doctor and the hospital should be part of the solution, rather than part of the problem.

And, of course, this being Alert Bay and Renee having been Indian while Dr. Pickup and the hospital administration are White, the issue couldn't help but be a racial one. In other words, the dispute wasn't being "turned into" a racial issue, it was *de facto* a racial issue. This had already been reflected, formally, in the fact that for the most part it had been Indians who had signed the petitions complaining about Dr. Pickup and non-Indians who had signed the petition in support of Dr. Pickup. Informally, the attitude of some people on the White End that it was inappropriate for *Indians* to complain about *Whites*, "after all they had done for them," had been expressed since Renee's death.

Some of Dr. Pickup's non-Indian supporters now began to accuse the Nimpkish Band Council of trying to capitalize on Renee's death in order to take over the hospital, a task they made it clear they thought Indians incapable of. These opinions were voiced publicly, vehemently and contemptuously. The attitudes they expressed were old ones which most Indians, regardless of their feelings about the issues at hand, recognized only too well. For some it was confirmation of what they'd always known: nothing had really changed over the years, the prejudice had simply become more subtle. For those who had believed that things really had changed, and had tried to convince others to forget old grievances, such responses were shocking and embarrassing.

The editor of the district's weekly newspaper, the *North Island Gazette*, published an editorial entitled "CURS SNAPPING AT THE HEELS OF AN OLD WARRIOR." Peter Paterson began with an effusive account of Dr. Pickup's career:

Back in 1953 there was no medicare in Canada....
That was the year Dr. Jack Pickup who delivered most of the babies

born in Alert Bay was having trouble with the Indian Health Services. They refused to pay the medical costs of any Indian except those legally declared to be indigent. Pickup was averaging $7 to $10 pay for each confinement, but he never turned an Indian mother away for lack of cash to pay the bill....

He had not always been a pilot. It was only after arriving in Alert Bay in 1949 and seeing how many people died or lost limbs needlessly because of the time it took them to reach medical care that Pickup took flying lessons, got his licence and bought a float plane.

Today it is 30 years later and Harold Pickup must be saying to himself, "I got to Alert Bay only yesterday, just a short while after my 30th birthday, where have all the years gone?"

They have gone by in a headlong torrent of emergency flights, middle of the night treatment of accident and brawling victims and the day by day grind of ministering to the medical needs of people who have been so displaced by an alien society that they seem almost possessed by an urge to physically self-destruct....

When it would have been easy and safe to play the bureaucrat and say nothing could be done; when lesser people would have shipped patients out to certain death in the fog of a two-day winter steamship trip to Vancouver, Pickup reached for a drill and did his best at backwoods, self-taught brain surgery, blood transfusions and all manner of risky emergency care.

People who shoulder the responsibility and do the tough jobs as best they can are the ones we all count on when we're in trouble. They are also the ones most vulnerable to attack by the mean in spirit.

Today, Dr. Pickup is the object of a particularly vicious attack.

It may be that he made a misjudgment which contributed to the eventual death of an 11-year-old girl who told a nurse trying to treat her, "I don't want to stay in this damn hospital." I don't know. I'm not competent to decide such a thing any more than any of the other local non-physicians, including those who have been spouting off to every radio, TV and daily newspaper reporter willing to give them some personal publicity....

It may be that the march of time with its air-sea rescue helicopters and daily jet flights to Vancouver has moved past the conditions in which Pickup dedicated himself as the round-the-clock, 365 days a year medical saviour of so many people for so many years.

It may be that the toll of thirty years of unrelenting medical labour is finally making itself felt....

I personally think that Harold Pickup is human like the rest of us and fallible, but he is also something more and that something is representative of the best and most noble qualities a human being can possess.

None of us is beyond question, but in light of his record those few who have instigated such a disproportionately furious attack upon Dr. Pickup must be either bursting with self-generated malice or lacking mental competence.

Response was immediate and vociferous, and the letters to the editor column of the *North Island Gazette* became a new forum for the debate. Band members voiced their opinions:

Sir:

As a member of the Nimpkish Indian Band who is neither "bursting with malice" nor "lacking in mental competence", I find your statements...curious to say the least....I consider you a "mostly new stranger", who has very little understanding of the situation, medical or otherwise, in Alert Bay....

—Gloria Cranmer Webster

Sir:

I am not speaking of the incident being investigated by the inquest alone but of the general conduct of Dr. Pickup in recent years....None of us has questioned the doctor's past history and at no time have our demands for an investigation been purposely vicious, as a matter of fact I think our conduct has been nothing but responsible.

Besides, as a people in a supposedly democratic society, we should have the right to speak out on any issue we find fault in and it appears there are 200 Indian "curs snapping" at the truth and if you and others like you can't understand this then all I can say is I feel a little sorry for you.

—George Speck Jr.

The students from the grades 4-6 class in the band's independent T'łisalagi'lakw School had their say, too:

Sir:

We think your article is very wrong. You are calling us down saying we are wild dogs and we are killing ourselves....You influence people into thinking doctors are super human. They aren't—neither are scientists or lawyers or nurses, etc. Doctors are supposed to help people—all peoples.

No one here "attacked" Dr. Pickup. People wanted to know how and why Renee died. Some of us were Renee's friends. We wanted to know too.

We think you should not put your prejudiced ideas in a public newspaper.

Others were cheekier:

Sir:

...An elder in my village once told me, 'The reason why most white people complain of pains in their neck is because they are always looking backwards.' Pickup may have been a great doctor in the past but that does not give him the right to practice medicine to-day if he is not capable.

—Wedledi Speck

And, not all band members agreed:

Sir:

As a resident of Alert Bay for 83 years, and as a member of the Nimpkish Indian Band, I feel obliged to comment on the controversy taking place in our village regarding the health situation and the criticism against Dr. Jack Pickup and the hospital.

I feel we should all be very proud of the hospital, and be thankful to have a doctor who has dedicated thirty-one years of his life here....

I am greatly disturbed at the allegations of the Nimpkish Band to the effect that Indians are being discriminated against and receiving substandard care. I find this impossible to accept when we not only have a hospital which...is above average, but also a government Indian service staffed by a registered nurse and two assistants.

I wish to go on record, as I stated to a C.B.C. reporter, but for some reason not reported, that I do not support the severe criticism of Dr. Pickup and the hospital and their demand for his immediate dismissal.

—Emma M. Kenmuir

A former resident of the area took issue specifically with Vera's report.

Sir:

Here is a copy of a letter I sent to the College of Physicians and Surgeons in Vancouver....

We lived in the surrounding isolated community from 1929 to 1963....I would like to say I have never met a doctor who was more dedicated to both the native and white population of Alert Bay and the isolated surrounding country that...[Dr. Pickup]...served so well....

The ratio of Indian deaths in relation to the whites was rather ridiculous considering more Indians than whites have been treated at Alert Bay Hospital through the years. Also in many cases their home life was detrimental to their health. I feel sure many of them would agree....

63

A wise chief once said, 'Do not condemn the Brave until you have walked in his moccasins.'
—Doris E. Murphy

And old friends and associates rallied to the doctor's defence:

Sir:

I am the Northern Supervisor for Gulf-Air Aviation and prior to that spent 14 years as pilot and operations manager for Alert Bay Air Services.... Dr. Pickup through sheer energy and devotion has managed to upgrade and initiate medical services in the area, and thus carve himself a place in the pioneering history of the North Coast.... [I] hope and pray that this great doctor's dignity, ability and devotion will...not be overshadowed by the preposterous charges laid against him by a couple of totally selfish, but very opinionated individuals followed by a flock of non-opinionated followers, who obviously enjoy all the attention created by such serious charges.... [Dr. Pickup] can personally take credit for the inter-island ferry system and the airstrip in Alert Bay which was constructed to improve the frequency of medical evacuations during bad weather conditions.... His kindness and concern for the native people in Alert Bay cannot be described by me.

Although I am convinced that Dr. Pickup's ability and standards will be appreciated by the...B.C. College of Physicians and Surgeons, it is, however, a fact that even totally cleared of all charges, the stigma shall always remain.... What a terrible injustice to a man who has totally dedicated his life to the medical services for the people of Alert Bay and the whole region.

How can this happen?
—Wm. (Villi) Douglas

Some questions were asked repeatedly by the urban-based reporters who arrived in town to cover the story, and by other "outsiders" who took an interest in the events: If the situation was as bad as the Indian representatives were claiming it was, and had been going on for as long as it apparently had, why had nothing been done about it before? How could the Indians have tolerated this for so many years? If these charges were true, and Renee's death was not an isolated incident, why then were some Indians defending Dr. Pickup and openly defying their own leaders? How could members of the St. George's Hospital Board of Trustees condone such a state of affairs? If the main problem was a drinking doctor, why was it being fought out as an Indians vs. Whites issue?

"Well," the answer usually came, "that's just the way it's always been around here. I guess you'd have to know Alert Bay to understand...."

64

CHAPTER 4

The Way It's Always Been Around Here

The problems we face here to-day go far beyond the practices of one local doctor. They date back one hundred years, to the way of thinking that characterizes non-Indian attitudes towards Indian people...
—Chief Roy Cranmer, Nimpkish Indian Band,
The Goldthorpe Inquiry (1980), Transcript Vol. 1, p. 70

No barbed wire separates the Village from the White End in Alert Bay. There are no guards at the ferry dock and no signs on public buildings. Generations of inter-marriage have produced some fair-haired children who cause hopeless confusion when they proudly volunteer to pose for tourists in front of totem poles. A visitor walking down Alert Bay's one main road on a summer day would encounter groups of women—from both ends of the island—talking and laughing as they push their baby carriages along. On the piers, fishermen, Indian and White, dressed identically in Stanfield shirts, blue jeans and gum boots, work on their nets, drink beer, and carry on a friendly banter. Looking past the docks to the mountains and the sea that surrounds the island, strangers are struck by the scenic beauty of the little town.

Most local people, if asked, would likely say that Indians and Whites in Alert Bay "get along pretty good most of the time." Nonetheless, Alert Bay is not one community. It is two. It always has been. Renee Smith was a child of one. Dr. Pickup is a pillar of the other.

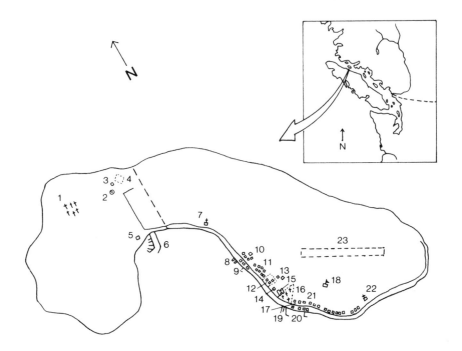

Nimpkish and Whe-La-La-U Indian Reserves

"The Village"

1. Graveyard
2. Totem Pole
3. Big House
4. Soccer Field
5. Old Residential School
6. Old Breakwater Dock

Municipality of Alert Bay

"The White End"

7. Anglican Church
8. Ferry Dock
9. Gas Dock, Shops, Drugstore
10. Hotel & Bar, Supermarket, Hardware Store
11. Firehall
12. R.C.M.P., Post Office, Liquor Store
13. Legion, Community Hall
14. Doctor's House
15. St. George's Hospital
16. Graveyard
17. Supermarket, Drygoods Store
18. School
19. Gas Dock, Shipyard
20. Hotel & Bar
21. Taxi, Movie Theatre
22. United Church
23. Airfield

For most urban Canadians, history is, perhaps, a personal interest, a curiosity. In rural, Indian/White communities like Alert Bay, history is an ever-present reality.

To understand the response to Renee's death in 1979, it is necessary to understand the history of Alert Bay.

I. IN THE BEGINNING

When the Transformer (or Creator), Ḵanikiʾlakw, travelled around the world, he eventually came to the place where Gwa'nalalis lived.

Ḵanikiʾlakw asked, "Would you like to become a cedar tree?"

Gwa'nalalis replied, "No, cedar trees, when struck by lightning, split and fall. Then they rot away for as long as the days dawn in the world."

Ḵanikiʾlakw asked again, "Would you like to become a mountain?"

"No," Gwa'nalalis answered. "For mountains have slides and crumble away for as long as the days dawn in the world."

The Transformer asked a third question. "Would you like to become a large boulder?"

Again, Gwa'nalalis answered, "No. Do not let me become a boulder, for I may crack in half and crumble away for as long as the days dawn in the world."

Finally, Ḵanikiʾlakw asked, "Would you like to become a river?"

"Yes, let me become a river that I may flow for as long as the days shall dawn in the world," Gwa'nalalis replied.

Putting his hand on Gwa'nalalis' forehead and pushing him down prone, Ḵanikiʾlakw said, "There friend, you will be a river and many kinds of salmon will come to you to provide food for your descendants for as long as the days shall dawn in the world."

And so, the man Gwa'nalalis became a river, Gwa'ni.

—legend of the origin of the Nimpkish River, original home of the Nimpkish people. Told by Pal'nakwala Wa'kas (Dan Cranmer), 1930, published by U'Mista Cultural Society.

According to their own origin legends, the Kwakwaka'wakw were placed in the central coast region of British Columbia by the Creator when time began.

According to archaeologists, the Kwakwaka'wakw are descendants of nomadic bands of hunter-fisher-gatherers who migrated across the Bering Bridge between Siberia and Alaska when the glaciers of the last Ice Age retreated, approximately 12,000 years ago.

For as long as anyone can remember, the Kwakwaka'wakw have used crescent-shaped Cormorant Island's natural bay as a refuge when storms interfere with travel on windy Johnstone Strait which separates Vancouver Island from the mainland. They call this haven 'Yalis, or "Spread Leg Beach," after the shape of the land formation which resembles a woman sitting on the beach with her legs spread open in front of her.

Commander George T. Gordon of the HMS *Cormorant*, a British warship employed to survey the B.C. coast in 1846, christened the island he claimed to have discovered "Cormorant Island." Twelve years later, in 1858, another warship, the HMS *Alert*, took shelter in "the small jewel which lay cradled in the arms of Cormorant Island"[1] and named the bay "Alert Bay."

The Kwakwaka'wakw were (are) a fishing people. The sea, and particularly the salmon who live(d) in it were (are) central to their existence. Deer, mountain goat, moose, bear and wild duck supplemented the many species of salmon, cod and shellfish which were (are) the staples of a rich and varied diet. Dense cedar forests offered huge planks and beams for multi-family Big Houses and canoes. Bark was stripped and used to make clothing, twine, baskets, nets and traps. Cedar logs were (are) transformed by skilled artists and craftsmen into elaborate totem poles and ornate ceremonial masks. Aboriginal social organization was (is) extremely complex as was (is) its central institution—the potlatch. For the purposes of this story, however, only the bare bones of the aboriginal system need be understood.

During the latter half of the nineteenth century European anthropologists, missionaries and administrators began compiling detailed, written reports about the Kwakwaka'wakw. These records describe the aboriginal Kwakwaka'wakw as having been organized into 'na'mima, each of which was founded by a mythical ancestor. 'Na'mima were (are) each headed by a chief and were (are) composed of several extended family groupings, or houses, and groups of 'na'mima formed larger units, or tribes, like the Nimpkish. Society was hierarchically organized into three main sectors: aristocrats, commoners and slaves. Noble rank is a hereditary status based on claims to direct descent from the original group of founding ancestors placed in the area by the Creator. Commoners were members of lineages whose founders could establish no such claims and slaves were members of neighbouring groups taken from their homes as captives of war.

The founding ancestors entered into pacts with the supernatural beings who controlled the land, the animals, the fish and other resources. In exchange for promising to demonstrate self-control, to share land and resources with others, to show proper respect for the animals, birds, fish and trees upon which human survival depends, and to pay appropriate homage to the supernatural owners of these riches, the ancestors were given the right to use these resources and to control their distribution among their people.

Chiefs organized their 'na'mima members in hunting, fishing, gathering, building and manufacture to meet both everyday subsistence needs and to produce surplus for redistribution at potlatches. The ability to accumulate large enough amounts of such surplus goods entitles a chief to give a potlatch and in so doing a chief and his 'na'mima fulfill their obligations to the ancestors and, through them, to the supernatural owners of the land. They re-affirm their hereditary rank, social position, and their right to govern by demonstrating generosity, displaying masks and crests, and in dance and song. Alliances are consolidated with other 'na'mima and villages, and disputes between individuals and groups are also settled at these gatherings. While these rituals are elaborate, the basic process is quite straightforward. A speaker states his or her case and people among the assembled guests having knowledge of the events either attest to, or deny, the validity of the speaker's account. Through this process, the truth is established and publicly confirmed and recorded.

Potlatches are held to announce, and record, births, marriages, deaths and other important occasions and were most frequently held during the winter months as summers were spent harvesting, processing and storing food. While noble rank is conferred at birth, failure to honour the obligations of rank can result in the leadership of a chief and his 'na'mima being challenged and overthrown.

Deaths from accidents and drowning were frequent, and infant mortality was high among the aboriginal Kwakwaka'wakw. However, abundant natural resources and well-developed food processing and storage techniques combined to ensure relatively good health for the population as a whole. Most adults had sufficient knowledge of a wide range of locally available herbal medicines to be able to take care of minor day-to-day problems, and children learned these skills as they grew up. The Kwakwaka'wakw followed a regimen of regular bathing in the ice cold sea and frequently took sweats to dispel bad feelings. As well as these healing practices, a whole host of rules and regulations that strictly governed the harvesting and preparation of food, the conduct of daily life, and major events such as childbirth, provided a cohesive preventive dimension to aboriginal health care.[2] Most fundamentally, good health was believed to lie in the strength of a person which, in turn, relied on the strength of the community.[3]

According to anthropologists, eighteenth and nineteenth century Kwakwaka'wakw believed in two types of illness. First, there was sickness caused by a loss of soul, or heart, for which the cure involved the recovery of the soul. Since the cause of such losses was usually attributed to the ill will of another person, the cure lay in the resolution of conflicts between people. Second, there were illnesses caused by more tangible disease objects which had, in some way or another, entered the body and which had to be removed.[4]

Responsibility for healing the sick in aboriginal society was essentially shared between two groups: shamans and elderly women. Shamans were believed to have obtained, from supernatural sources, power over life and death which allowed them to either cause illness or to cure it. Both the shamans and the elderly women who were healers, employed a combination of natural medicines, prayer, ritual and personal counselling—what we would now call psychotherapy—in their treatments. Healers, however, were not seen as possessing the same degree of supernatural power as the shamans. They could cure, but not cause, disease. Shamans and healers alike treated both sorts of illnesses, sometimes working together and sometimes individually. Features common to all healing practices were their public nature and the required attendance of the elders of the village at curing ceremonies.[5] Surrounding the patient with social support was considered essential to the healing process.

Wielding control over life and death is a source of power in all societies, and Kwakwaka'wakw shamans were influential men who figured very prominently in the aboriginal political structure. Shamans were members of the nobility who were said to have been "owned by the chiefs" and to have been frequently ordered to kill the chiefs' enemies by "throwing" disease into them. Future shamans were selected at a young age, given intensive training and subjected to gruelling initiations into secret societies after which they were forbidden for at least four years from asking for payment for their services and were expected, instead, to accept whatever compensation patients thought them worthy of. Once he had proven himself, a successful shaman could set his own price.[6]

Powerful as the shamans, who held names like "Life-Owner," "Making-Alive" and "Life Brought Out Of Canoe," were, their power held sway only as long as they could produce either tangible proof of their abilities or plausible explanations for their failures. If a patient died while in the care of a shaman, the shaman was expected to compensate the deceased's family for their loss. A shaman who lost too many patients or whose cures were found to be ineffective could be declared a fraud, or could be suspected of being in the employ of a rival chief, and could thus find himself impoverished, with neither patients nor chiefly patrons to support him.[7]

The first recorded European contact with the Kwakwaka'wakw was the arrival of Captain George Vancouver in 1792, who described his visit to a village at the mouth of the Nimpkish River, located directly across Johnstone Strait from Alert Bay, as follows:

> The houses, in number 34, were arranged in regular streets; the larger ones were the habitations of the principal people, who had them decorated with paintings and other ornaments, forming various figures....The women were variously employed; some in their different household affairs, others in the manufacture of their garments from bark and other materials, the fabrication of mats for a variety of purposes, and a kind of basket, wrought so curiously close as to contain water like an earthen vessel without the least leakage or drip,

comprehended the general employment of the women, who were not less industrious than ingenious.[8]

The Kwakwaka'wakw became actively involved in the fur trade during the first half of the nineteenth century and in 1849, the Hudson's Bay Company established Fort Rupert in the central Kwakwaka'wakw area. To the Kwakwaka'wakw, the new opportunities for trade and the increasing availability of European manufactured goods provided an opportunity for the elaboration of the central institution of aboriginal society: the potlatch. Potlatches became more frequent and access to, and the ability to accumulate, large amounts of European goods became a determining factor in achieving rank. During the fur trade era, such an elaboration of the potlatch did not directly conflict with the objectives of the Europeans, who were clearly interested in trade rather than in settlement. Ships' logs and journals kept by traders testify to the fact that Native peoples on the Northwest Coast exercised significant control over the trade by such means as withholding furs to drive up prices, placing "advance orders" for specific trade goods, and refusing to trade unless satisfied with the goods being offered in exchange.[9]

The latter half of the nineteenth century brought with it the collapse of the European and Asian fur markets and, consequently, the decline of the fur trade. This corresponded to the advent of the Gold Rush and the beginning of intensive and permanent European settlement on the B.C. coast. These years mark the period during which the basic colonial structures that continue to shape the relationship between Euro-Canadians and Native peoples came into being. On the B.C. coast, as elsewhere, the decimation of the aboriginal population by epidemic diseases brought by Europeans played a major role in establishing the foundations of this relationship. Indigenous peoples found themselves rapidly becoming minorities in their own lands, and while a certain degree of economic independence could be maintained by continuing to live off the land, social demoralization, sickness, and dependence on European medical care to cure European diseases began to take their toll.[10]

As early as 1787 epidemics of smallpox, influenza and measles had been recorded among the Native populations of B.C. However, with more and more Indians travelling to trading forts and camping around new cities like Victoria, these contagious diseases, against which the Indians had neither natural immunity nor effective medicine, began to threaten their very existence. Anthropologist Wilson Duff offers the following description of the smallpox epidemic of 1862:

Following upon the first gold excitement in 1858, it became the habit of many northern coastal tribes to visit Victoria in larger numbers and at times, more than 2000 'Hydahs', 'Stickeens', 'Chimseans', 'Bella Bellas', 'Fort Ruperts', and so on were camped on the outskirts of the settlement. That was the situation in April, 1862, when a white man with smallpox arrived from San Francisco. Before long, despite dire warnings in the 'Colonist', the disease reached the camps of the Indians and they began to die in fearful numbers. Alarmed, the authorities burned the camps and forced the Indians to leave.

They started up the Coast for home, taking the disease with them, leaving the infection at every place they touched. The epidemic spread like a forest fire up the coast and into the Interior.[11]

The epidemics had a dramatic impact on aboriginal society as the possibility of imminent and total extinction became a very real one. What medical relief was available was provided by missionaries who, as they did in other parts of the world, arrived following the worst ravages of the colonial encounter, offering medicine, salvation and hope to desperate peoples. A Haida Chief, talking to one of these early missionaries, told him:

Our people are brave in warfare and never turn their backs on their foes, but this foe we could not see and we could not fight. Our medicine men are wise, but they could not drive away the evil spirit, and why? Because it was the sickness of the Iron People. It came from them.[12]

The first census taken of the Kwakwaka'wakw was conducted by John Work around 1835 and he estimated the total population to be around 10,700. Fifty years later, in 1885, this figure had dropped by approximately 72 per cent, to around 3000.[13]

The new settlers who began arriving in droves after 1850, unlike the transient fur traders who preceded them, were interested in acquiring ownership of land and resources and, to a degree, in exploiting indigenous labour. Therefore we find, in the accounts of the early settlers, aboriginal life no longer described as "industrious and ingenious" but rather as lazy, immoral and brutal:

...shall we allow a few vagrants to prevent forever industrious settlers from settling on the unoccupied lands? Not at all. Locate reservations for them on which to earn their own living, and if they trespass on white settlers punish them severely. A few lessons would soon enable them to form a correct estimation of their own inferiority, and settle the Indian title too!

Editorial, *Victoria British Colonist*, 1861:3

...according to the strict rule of international law territory occupied by a barbarous or wholly uncivilized people may be rightfully appropriated by a civilized or Christian nation.

The British Columbian, June 1, 1869:5

II. THE WHITE MAN'S BURDEN

The people who founded Alert Bay's White community did not arrive on the shores of Cormorant Island completely unprepared. Like the Kwakwaka'wakw, Europeans and Euro-Canadians had a particular understanding of how their world worked. Like the Kwakwaka'wakw, they too had children and grandchildren to whom they passed on their possessions and their knowledge. They too welcomed newcomers into their community over the years and taught them how to live with their neighbours.

The settlers, missionaries and administrators who flooded into British Columbia were men and women who were seeking to establish secure and productive lives under circumstances and in conditions entirely unknown to their parents. While some came from European countries, and others from as far away as Hawaii and China, most were immigrants from England, or descendants of earlier waves of British immigrants who had settled in Eastern Canada. So it is to the Britain of the late nineteenth and early twentieth centuries that Alert Bay's White community proudly traces its roots.

By the latter half of the nineteenth century rapid industrialization at home and colonial expansion abroad had brought dramatic changes to Great Britain since the early years of that century when fur-trading companies initially became involved with the Kwakwaka'wakw. Accompanying these economic and political developments were new understandings of inequality at home, and of the differences between Europeans and the aboriginal peoples they encountered in colonies all over the world.

The discovery by Charles Darwin of scientific evolution driven by the law of natural selection—or survival-of-the-fittest—in the plant and animal world, had profound effects on European attitudes when it was applied to questions of human behaviour and inequality. Theories concerning social evolution were particularly influential among British and American anthropologists, who, in turn, supplied explanations to the public as to the character of the differences between colonizing and colonized peoples.

Simply put, nineteenth-century evolutionism—or Social Darwinism, as one of these schools of thought came to be called—attempted to explain the history of the human race, and variation among its branches, by means of a model borrowed from biology. Using the chronology of European history—such as agriculture having followed pastoralism and hunting-gathering, and industrial capitalism having followed feudalism—as their model, evolutionists asserted that these constituted universal stages of development passed through, at varying rates, by the whole human race. Evolutionists arranged these stages on a ladder, and claimed that each represented an advance in technology, morality, government and intelligence. By following this logic, social scientists surmised that Western European, upper middle class males—which, coincidentally, most of them happened to be—obviously represented the pinnacle of human evolutionary achievement.

Of major importance in this belief system was the relationship between evolution and human intelligence. People who celebrated private ownership of delineated plots of land were considered to be thinking more abstractly, and were therefore presumed to be more intelligent, than those who supported group ownership. Individuals who placed personal ambition and the acquisition of material goods highest on their list of goals were assumed to be thinking more rationally, and were more fully evolved, than those who displayed more concern for families and traditions, or who spent their money fulfilling social obligations. While within each group there were those who were seen as more or less intelligent, even the lowliest member of a superior group was considered at least a touch more developed—having reached a higher stage of evolution—than the most advanced member of an inferior group. This framework provided the basis for explaining inequality between men and women, between classes, and between national and racial groups.

The reports of missionaries, Indian Agents and settlers are rife with the crudest interpretations of Social Darwinism.[14] William Halliday, who, in the course of his forty-odd years in the Kwakwaka'wakw area, from 1896 to 1935, was a settler, a lay missionary, an Indian Agent, and a residential school principal, published his memoirs. In them he offers the following analysis of local evolutionary developments and an insight into the principles that guided him in his work.

> Possibly another reason may be given why the Indians physique is improving, but the reason does not reflect creditably on the white people. It is owing to the infusion of white blood that these results are occurring. A very large percentage of the Indians to-day are not of pure Indian blood, and, as one can imagine, it is not the better class of white men who have thus degraded themselves by intermingling with the Indian women, so that the result morally is not so great as the result physically. However, it will hasten the time when Indians as such will be no more, but will be absorbed into the white race, and will help to carry the burden that so far has been borne by the white man for his benefit.[15]

In Europe, the rule of monarchs and aristocrats was gradually usurped as kings, noblemen and peasants were replaced by elected politicians, bureaucrats, wealthy industrialists, wage labourers, and displaced peasants, and the foundations of the modern liberal democracies of countries such as Canada were laid. The ideology—or, some would say, mythology—of liberal democracy rests on the assumption that modern western societies, rather than being governed by tradition, custom and inherited privilege and power, are more justly governed by the democratic election of leaders who, like others who are successful in such a society, achieve their positions on the basis of individual merit, ability and hard work.

As the Industrial Revolution gathered momentum in Britain vast numbers of peasants were forced off their lands and into the cities where some found employment in workshops and factories, while others found themselves reduced to begging, crime and prostitution. Betwixt and between the old aristocracy, the captains of industry, the displaced peasants and the industrial workers was a new and growing middle class consisting of small businessmen, doctors, managers, artisans, educators, academics, scientists, clerics and other professionals whose wealth and power lay as much in their knowledge and technical expertise as in their heritage. Of this group, many were appalled by the living conditions of the poor that they saw before them and by the brutal indifference to such suffering displayed by those in power. They feared that the combination of wanton greed and cruelty on the part of the wealthy classes, and the dismal ignorance and immorality of the poorer classes, would lead to the disintegration of their society.

Such social reformers advocated legislative changes such as child labour laws to alleviate the worst ravages of industrialization, and public works projects to improve urban living conditions. They founded philanthropic organizations to give assistance to the poor and to teach them to improve their lives by developing the virtues of industriousness, frugality, temperance, and cleanliness. The necessary foundation to this approach to social reform is, of course, the belief that a major obstacle to success is lack of individual ability or ambition. Philanthropy had the effect of seeming to ameliorate the unhappy conditions of the poor without challenging the fundamental organization of power in society. In addition, the belief that the principles and methods of natural science could be used to manage society and to transform and discipline human populations to adapt to new social orders gained prominence and contributed to the popularity of experiments in social engineering and eugenics.

Therefore we find during this period of European history the growing importance of two institutions whose very nature embodies the contradiction described above: public education and public health. Both were demanded as reforms to improve the lives of the disadvantaged. Both were organized around the basic assumption that their task was to address a two-fold problem.

On the one hand the poor had been denied the necessary training, or treatment, that would allow them to improve their lot and this situation was to be rectified by making such training and/or treatment available to them. On the other hand, the poor had habits, values, life-styles and often a lack of intellectual development, that contributed to ill health and high mortality rates and that prevented them from taking advantage of opportunities to better themselves. This, too, was to be rectified by treatment, training and, if necessary, by punishment.

In the field of medicine and health care, professional experts, trained in specialized institutions, claimed exclusive ownership of the knowledge and techniques required to save lives and heal the sick while also assuming the political role of "guardians of public morals and public health alike."[16] A necessary qualification for entry into the medical profession, therefore, became not only scientific training in the diagnosis and treatment of disease, but also membership in an elite sector of society charged with maintaining and enforcing the established order.

One of the major obstacles to the development of the medical profession's exclusive jurisdiction over the human body was the knowledge and skill in the practice of folk medicine possessed by many non-professionals, frequently women. Many of these healers and their remedies were outlawed, some were declared witches and executed, and all efforts were made to prevent them from passing their knowledge on to subsequent generations. In the context of European colonization of the Northwest Coast, it was the power of shamans and the knowledge of aboriginal medicines which had to be undermined to accomplish this goal. The onslaught of the epidemics and the inability of indigenous healers to cure the victims accelerated this process.

It was this British society of the Victorian era, with its obsessive faith in science and progress, and its equally unshakeable confidence in its own inherent superiority, that produced the colonial administrators, the missionaries, and many of the settlers who came to the coast of British Columbia during the latter half of the nineteenth century and the early years of the twentieth century.

As industry flourished, the need for both raw materials and new markets pushed Britain further into colonial adventures. British Columbia was a land rich in natural resources and a railway was being built which would connect British North America from coast to coast and to ports serving Europe, Asia and the ever-prospering United States. The land had to be brought under the control of the Empire, and who better to perform the labour of logging, mining, fishing and homesteading than those thousands of workers and displaced farmers congregating in potentially disruptive numbers in over-crowded cities in Europe and Eastern Canada. For some, the promise of employment, or greater religious freedom and personal independence was sufficient motivation to voluntarily emigrate. There is land and gold for the taking and plenty for all, they were told. You are civilized, you are Christian and you are white. The savages have been contained and should pose no insurmountable problems.

For administrators, assignment to the colonies was in some cases a punishment for wrong-doing, in some cases a convenient means of respectably disposing of errant sons, and in some cases the fulfillment of a Christian-imperialist mission. Individuals with all these various motivations and combinations thereof found themselves in the colonial service where their tasks were to secure land for settlement and resources for commerce, and to maintain law, order and civilization.

Missionaries, on the other hand, were more single-minded. Many were radicals within their own churches, fundamentalists who disapproved of the

76

pomp, glamour and power displayed by members of the religious hierarchies, and who were horrified by the decadence and debauchery of the idle rich. For them the "New World" offered an opportunity to truly create the Kingdom of Heaven on earth—or at least within the British Empire. Indians, while generally regarded as backward savages, were also seen as children of nature, unsullied and uncorrupted by the evils of industrial civilization. The missionaries envisioned themselves living simple lives, close to the land, creating communities based on agriculture and cottage industries in little isolated villages which would be havens of purity and perfection. Christian virtues and British ideals would be planted in simple minds where they could be nourished and cultivated, safely protected from the temptations of greed and worldly ambition.

III. ONWARD CHRISTIAN SOLDIERS

My first operation was to open a day-school. So the battle began. My pupils were my infantry. Few or many, I drudged away daily at A, B, C, and 1, 2, 3.

Now I must describe my artillery practice. The medicine chest is my ammunition tumbrel. Stoppered phials have been my Armstrong guns, and my shells were hurled on the foe from pill boxes. During school hours bodies of wounded would accumulate, and, school over, my artillery would be plied. Five hundred and fifty applications for healing have been made, and if, as the medicine-men say, I have killed some, I have relieved so many that I am the most famous medicine-man known to the nation.

So raged the battle.

—William Ridley, Missionary, 1881[17]

Well, a war is not a war unless both sides are fighting, and while British Columbia did not experience armed rebellions on the scale of those fought during the settlement of the American West, the indigenous peoples of the Northwest Coast neither welcomed colonization with open arms, nor were they bowled over by an eminently superior civilization. Rather, they sought, as they still do to-day, a rational, fair, and mutually beneficial agreement with the new occupants of their lands.

The first official land confiscations in B.C. were those effected in 1864 by Joseph Trutch, colonial land commissioner, who justified the seizures on the grounds that Indians were "utter savages" incapable of understanding "abstract" ideas of property. Trutch allotted land to Indians on the basis of ten acres per family. Homesteading settlers were given, officially, 160 acres each. In 1874, and again in 1880, British Columbia Natives in vain protested these allotments by means of petitions to the colonial authorities.

As the new industries of commercial fishing, canning and logging opened up along the coast, Native people eagerly sought employment in them. Their knowledge, ability and industriousness, particularly in fishing, made them a highly skilled and desirable labour force, especially during the latter half of the nineteenth century when Natives still out-numbered non-Natives in the provincial population, despite the effects of the epidemics. However, continued access to subsistence from the land and sea made the wages Natives earned largely what we now call "disposable income," i.e. income not required for the necessities of life. As during the fur trade, new sources of wealth and European goods were quickly incorporated into aboriginal society and used to elaborate the potlatch system. This posed problems for pioneer entrepreneurs, including those who settled in Alert Bay. Their successors tell the story as follows:

> The original white settlers of Alert Bay were two intrepid pioneers who came overland across the Isthmus of Panama and up the coast in a sailing sloop....
>
> [T]he two partners...leased Cormorant Island from the government, and established a settlement. Here, they constructed in 1870 a small saltery, salting and mild-curing salmon which were sent mostly to Victoria.
>
> Spencer and Huson...had trouble with the Indians as employees. They did not believe in work for work's sake. At the slightest provocation, such as a wedding, potlatch, or similar, they would sail off home or on a visit to neighbouring clans. It must be remembered that in the days before the coming of the white man, the Indian did not have what we call an occupation...He required no money as we have, as there was nothing to purchase. His food was to his hand whenever he needed it. It was a pleasure to fish or hunt and the "klootch", his wife, dried the fish and made the cake and cared for the children....
>
> At first, the Indian did not take kindly to steady work, but...he more or less got used to being called upon to work against his natural preference.
>
> The transition was a slow process and Spencer and Huson were anxious for the sake of their business to try and hurry it along a bit. So the two partners conceived the idea of founding an Indian village near their plant and persuading the Nimpkish River Indians to move their homes to Alert Bay. With this in mind they approached Reverend Alfred James Hall, a missionary of the Church Missionary Society.... These two enterprising young men prevailed upon Mr. Hall to move his mission to Alert Bay by promising to build a mission house for him....
>
> Mr. Hall succumbed to their persuasions and moved to Alert Bay in 1878.[18]

While the fundamental objective of colonizers has always been to expropriate the land, resources and labour of indigenous peoples, the particular methods used to accomplish this goal have varied throughout the world over many centuries and have been conditioned by differences in geography and climate, in economy, in culture, and in the social and political organization of both colonizing powers and indigenous societies. In Canada, for example, the Newfoundland Beothuks were massacred *en masse* by colonial settlers in the seventeenth and eighteenth centuries. The aboriginal peoples of Eastern Canada were pressed into military service in the colonial wars fought between Britain, France and the American Colonies. During the nineteenth century, the buffalo herds which the Plains Cree depended upon were wiped out, thereby making land available for the agricultural development of the Prairies.

The colonization of the British Columbia coast bears the indelible stamp of Victorian England. The influence of nineteenth-century philanthropic and social engineering movements in Britain was reflected in a colonial policy which has been described by the historian John Tobias as one based on the principles of "protection, civilization and assimilation."[19] The assumptions of policy makers were that Indians would be "protected" from evil and immoral sectors of the white population who it was felt both took advantage of the "simple" Natives and who furthermore set a bad example. They would be "civilized" by being educated in British beliefs and life-styles by Victorian missionaries, and the result would be the transformation of future generations into Euro-Canadians—"assimilation." In other words, it was assumed that Native peoples would cease to exist as distinct, identifiable cultures either capable or desirous of maintaining ownership of their land or resources, or of resisting the dominant order in any other way. Resistance, or lack of co-operation, was interpreted as an inability or unwillingness to adapt to a superior way of life, and this in itself constituted evidence of either biological or cultural inferiority, or both.

These principles were embodied in the establishment of reserves and in the Indian Act of 1876, which brought virtually every aspect of Native life under government administration. This included, for the Kwakwaka'wakw, confinement to reserves under the direct surveillance of government agents, compulsory education by missionaries, the prohibition of alcohol, and, in 1884, the banning of the potlatch. In 1890 the Kwakiutl Agency of the Department of Indian Affairs established its administrative headquarters at Alert Bay and the British Columbia Provincial Police stationed their first full-time constable there, thus making Alert Bay the economic, administrative, educational and religious centre of the colonial regime within the Kwakwaka'wakw region.

It was the continued predominance of the potlatch in Kwakwaka'wakw life, however, which most frustrated the ambitions of missionaries, administrators, and settlers alike. Not only were potlatches offensive to the Protestant Ethic but they were also the forums in which the indigenous land tenure system was perpetuated by means of the passing on from one generation to the next, through names, ownership and rights to land and resources. It was also at potlatches that marriages, births and deaths were publicly recorded and legitimated and where the young were taught traditional codes of behaviour and morality. Thus, the existence of the potlatch ran counter to assimilationist goals at their very core.

As they fought for land and resource ownership rights, Native peoples up and down the coast also protested the criminalization of potlatching by way of petitions to the authorities, letters to the editors of provincial newspapers, appeals to sources of power, and outright defiance. As late as 1921, thirty-seven years after clauses banning the potlatch had been added to the Indian Act, Nimpkish Chief Dan Cranmer, of Alert Bay, hosted his now famous potlatch at the neighbouring village of Mamallilikala. The R.C.M.P. raided the potlatch; participants were arrested; masks, screens, coppers and other "potlatch paraphernalia" were confiscated and forty-five people served jail terms in Oakalla Prison for having participated. Potlatching, nevertheless, continued secretly in the more isolated Kwakwaka'wakw villages and in Alert Bay itself.

Struggle as they might, the Kwakwaka'wakw found the cards stacked against them in their bid for autonomous co-existence with their new neighbours. In 1906 and 1909 delegations of B.C. Chiefs carried their grievances to London. From 1912 to 1916 the McKenna-McBride Joint Royal Commission on Indian Affairs in British Columbia toured the province. Chiefs presented documented evidence of their needs regarding the size and scope of reserve land acreage as well as hunting and fishing rights. In reply, the Royal Commission reduced the size of the existing reserves.

In 1916, B.C. Indians organized themselves under the banner of the Allied Tribes of British Columbia for the purposes of presenting their land claims directly to the British Privy Council. In 1927, a Joint Federal/Provincial Committee responded to the demands put forward by the Allied Tribes of B.C. by outlawing the formation of political organizations, the calling of meetings, and the raising of funds for the purposes of pursuing Native land claims.

This era also witnessed the beginnings of institutionalized medical care in B.C., and with it a pattern of relationships which still persists to-day. Since the early years of this century, British Columbia doctors have been disproportionately represented in political leadership positions from the local to the provincial level and have figured prominently as investors in the province's economy. In other words, in the socio-economic structure of British Columbia, doctors have consistently occupied the highest ranking positions in terms of economic privilege and social prestige, while Indians have been relegated to the lowest positions.

Dr. I. W. Powell, of United Empire Loyalist stock, assumed ownership of huge tracts of land in the province's lower mainland, and was appointed the first Superintendent of Indian Affairs for the Province of British Columbia in 1872. Medical historians pay tribute to this man in their accounts of the development of their profession:

> Dr. Powell's energetic life of service in medicine, politics, education, military and Indian affairs was in a way typical of early physicians who became leaders in many areas outside their own field of expertise.[20]

But Dr. Rose, a physician and historian of the B.C. medical profession, admits that not all of B.C.'s early doctors were noble pioneers:

> With few exceptions, the impulse to traverse a wilderness and practice under primitive conditions was obeyed largely by men who realized that they were not likely to achieve distinction in more urbane and academic centres....[21]
> Conscientious doctors often visited each of their charges twice a month...travelling as much as thirty miles a day by horse...There were others who spent their time lying drunk, and in some remote and unprofitable areas sick men were brutally neglected.[22]

In 1886 the provincial legislature passed into law the Medical Act which established the British Columbia College of Physicians and Surgeons, whose mandate was to establish and enforce rules and regulations to govern the licensing and disciplining of medical practitioners. The intention was to guarantee uniform and quality medical care to the province's population.

While scientific research and professional regulation have contributed to advances in technology and medicine which have served the human race well, these developments have not taken place in a social vacuum. Technology and knowledge are utilized by particular people in particular environments, and it is often the context in which medicine is practised, rather than the sophistication of medical theory or techniques, that determines its effectiveness. The following comparison, written by a British Columbia doctor and medical historian, of differences between aboriginal medical care and that practised by European and Euro-Canadian medical professionals, attests to this fact—somewhat ironically in the context of the story being told here.

> The health care system of the coastal Indians, remarkable as it was, was handicapped by the absence of a written language. All knowledge, medical and otherwise, was handed down by word of mouth from one generation to the next. This verbal method of passing on information lacked the cumulative power of the written word which, particularly in medicine, permits painstaking comparisons that result

in progressively constructive diagnostic and therapeutic refinements.

The Indian's method of recording a significant event was to weave a legend about it....

Thus, there were a number of legends that were used empirically for the eradication of the bad spirits that caused an illness classified comprehensively as 'pains in the stomach.' It was left to the luck of the sick Indian as to whether the legend chosen for his cure dealt with the ailment from which he actually suffered. One can easily picture the catastrophic result of treating according to a 'pain in the stomach' legend suitable for gall bladder disease a patient actually afflicted with acute appendicitis.[23]

The demographic balance between Indians and non-Indians in B.C. had shifted by the 1920s, and the Kwakwaka'wakw population reached its lowest point—1,834 persons—in 1929. This figure represents approximately 15 per cent of the size of the pre-contact population, or an 85 per cent decrease in barely one hundred years. While the smallpox epidemics that raged throughout the years from 1837 to 1880 had claimed most of these lives, smallpox was replaced by measles, venereal disease, tuberculosis and influenza, whose combined effects continued to take their toll.

TABLE 1[24]

Population Decline and Growth: British Columbia, 1835–1980

Year	Kwakwaka'wakw	B.C.Indians	B.C.Non-Indians
1835	10,700	70,000	unknown
1885	3,000	28,000	15,000
1929	1,834	22,605	694,300
1949	1,961	27,936	1,200,000
1961	2,500	38,914	1,398,500
1980	3,648	57,759	2,571,200

While Indian Agents dispensed medicines supplied by the federal government, it was missionaries, like those who travelled to both Native villages and isolated logging camps on the Anglican Church medical missionary boat, the *Columbia*, who were largely responsible for administering medical care to the Kwakwaka'wakw.

The Anglican Church financed the building of a hospital at nearby Rock Bay in 1905. This hospital was, however, a "Whites Only" institution. The Kwakwaka'wakw therefore welcomed the construction of the first St. George's Hospital in Alert Bay in 1909, which was financed by the B.C. Packers Fishing Company, the provincial government, the Indian Department, the

Women's Auxiliary to Missions of the Church of England in Canada, and by the Kwakwaka'wakw. Having no word in the Kwa'kwala language for such an institution, the Indians called *ts'aka'atsi* which means "a container for the sick." The original building burned down in 1923 and was rebuilt and reopened in 1925 amidst much pomp and ceremony:

> On May 13, 1925 the hospital was formally opened by Major Selden Humphries, DSO, ADC, representing the Lieutenant-Governor. The Columbia arrived . . . carrying Bishop Schoefield . . . and Archdeacon Heathcote.
>
> One hundred cadets of the Indian industrial school, girls of the Indian Girls' Home and the Indian saxophone band welcomed them ashore, where Welcome and *Hamatsa* dances were performed for them by the Indians. Chief Whonnock of Fort Rupert said in his speech, "This hospital is to us the house of salvation and the house of hope. Salvation for the present and hope for the generations to come."
>
> Later, the *Columbia* called at reserves at Village Island and Alert Bay where...sacks of money totalling $1500 were presented to Antle. The money, a large sum for those days, was donated for an X-ray machine for the hospital. The Indians felt this was their special institution. Indians and whites were in separate wards, but the mission went to great lengths to give equal service to both.[25]

The stringent enforcement of the anti-potlatch law; increased pressure from missionaries, governments, and law enforcement agencies to surrender children to educational institutions; a recession in the logging and fishing industries; and continuing sickness and high mortality, made the 1920s a painful period in Kwakwaka'wakw history. While missionaries and settlers congratulated themselves on having won the battle against the forces of Satan, Kwakwaka'wakw anthropologist Gloria Cranmer Webster later described this era as follows:

> Schools and hospitals moved in on our people when we were most vulnerable. In the early part of this century, we really did appear to be a 'vanishing race'.[26]

IV. ALERT BAY 1930-1969

From wilderness peopled by native tribes, the Alert Bay district has grown to contain thriving industries and prosperous businesses...
Its beginnings were humble, but the hard work, ingenuity, and faith in its future that constituted the makeup of her pioneers made Alert Bay

No longer just a small enclave of administrators, cannery owners and missionaries, Alert Bay's White community grew and diversified from 1930 through the '40s, '50s and '60s. Transient fishermen, loggers and miners continued to pass through but more began to stay. Most continued to earn their living from fishing and logging, while others opened small businesses like shipyards, cafes, hotels and bars, dry goods stores, taxis and grocery outlets. Some married Native women and since the Indian Act deprived women of their legal status as Indians when they married non-Indians, thereby prohibiting them from living on reserves, these families established a "mixed" community on the "White End" of town where they raised their children.

The Alert Bay area's reputation as a hard-workin', hard-drinkin', hard-fightin', hard-lovin' frontier society was formed during this era. This image of a rugged pioneer past is cultivated with pride by local non-Natives.[27]

Native men worked as commercial fishermen and loggers alongside non-Natives. However, when they gambled, drank or spent their wages on recreation along with their non-Indian cohorts, rather than being seen as a demonstration of vigorous masculinity, such behaviour was considered evidence of an inability to plan and save, a childish obsession with frivolous amusements, and an irresponsible attitude towards their families. Indian legal and political rights were determined by their position as wards of the state, still undergoing "training" to prepare them for "civilization." Administration and surveillance of every detail of Indian life from birth, education, marriage, homemaking, child-rearing, health, occupation, movement on and off the reserve, business dealings, deaths, funerals, last wills and testaments and the disposal of estates was carried on by Indian Agents under the auspices of the Indian Act.

An Anglican-administered industrial residential school, St. Michael's, which housed upwards of 200 students, was established in Alert Bay in1929. Attendance was compulsory, and the Indian Act provided for a variety of punishments which could be levied against unco-operative parents, including fines and jail sentences. Students were prohibited from speaking their own language, and along with training in Christian scriptures and a basic academic program up to a grade 8 level, boys were taught carpentry, mechanics, farming, and animal husbandry, while girls received instruction in cooking, sewing and homemaking.

The explicit goal of the residential school system was to break the bonds between generations, thus "freeing" the young from the shackles of tradition and the influence of their families. Native parents, of course, made every effort to thwart this estrangement from their children and more and more people migrated from the smaller, more isolated Kwakwaka'wakw villages to Alert Bay in order to be able, at least, to visit with their children regularly. For the most part graduates of the residential schools did not assimilate into Canadian society. Many had no desire to, and others who tried found the doors closed to them. At the same time, when they returned to their home villages they often found they had lost both the ability to communicate fluently with parents and grandparents, and the practical, as well as social, skills necessary to fit into village life.[28]

While rank and social status determined by the potlatch system continued to function within Kwakwaka'wakw society, new divisions rooted in colonial relations arose and either overlapped with the aboriginal hierarchy or co-existed beside it. The terms and conditions for survival and opportunities for upward mobility—often synonymous terms in this context—were now defined by the dominant non-Native society and were therefore most available to Native people who possessed one or more of the following attributes: conversion to Christianity, mission or residential school education, at least formal denunciation of potlatching and other elements of aboriginal culture, mixed blood, and residence in Alert Bay rather than in one of the outlying villages. Some Indians did become successful skippers or boat owners in the commercial fishing industry and a few found steady work in logging. Others owned and ran small stores on the reserves. The majority, however, worked when work was available and/or received government relief.

The health of the Kwakwaka'wakw population began a slow but steady improvement during the 1930s. Tuberculosis now rivalled measles, influenza and venereal disease as the main health problem and cause of death among B.C. Indians, and a T.B. Preventorium was built on the grounds of St. Michael's. Prolonged stays in hospitals and sanitoriums became a normal part of life for many Kwakwaka'wakw, while the ever-increasing dependency of Native people on the medical profession came to be taken for granted by patients, doctors and hospital staff alike. By the end of the 1930s, most of the Kwakwaka'wakw living in Alert Bay had converted to Christianity, and education, rather than being resisted, began to be encouraged for the young.

"We had to think about what will be best for the kids," a Kwakwaka'wakw elder would later explain.[29]

The 1940s brought with them a number of significant developments in relations between Alert Bay's two communities. The economic boom initiated by World War II stimulated the logging industry, and the exclusion of the Japanese from commercial fishing by internment and relocation created advantages for both Native and non-Native fishermen. The Pacific Coast Native Fisherman's Association, formed by Alert Bay fishermen during the 1930s, amalgamated with the Native Brotherhood of B.C. in 1945. The executive of the new organization contained several Native boat-owners from Alert Bay. Non-Native union fishermen and Native non-union fishermen formed the two major groups on the coast, and among the fishermen of Alert Bay.

The Native Brotherhood did not confine its activities to the fishing industry, but lobbied as well for civil rights, improved health care and increased educational opportunities for Indians. When the Second World War was declared many Kwakwa̱ka'wakw men signed up and fought overseas. New bitternesses developed when they came home and still could not vote, could not drink, and could not join the Legion. Antagonism was further exacerbated by the fact that Indian fishermen had agreed to pay income tax for the first time to contribute to the war effort, had paid substantial taxes on their relatively high wages, and had then been informed, after the war ended, that they would be required to continue paying income taxes—despite the fact that they were not citizens.

The post-World War II era is noted by many analysts as a turning point in Indian/White relations. Following the defeat of Hitler and the revelations of Nazi atrocities, the western world entered a period of racial liberalism. Canada's image of itself, both nationally and internationally, as a free, democratic country where all citizens are equal regardless of race, colour or creed, was marred by the existence of a category of people whose legal, political and social existence was defined by their "race." Indians became a source of public embarrassment and efforts began to be made to improve living conditions on reserves and, once again, to assimilate Indians into mainstream Canadian society. Federal government funding was increased, particularly in the areas of health care and education. As one local man described this period of time,

> It just seemed like white people started to realize that what they'd done to the Indians all these years—keeping us in the dark like that—it was wrong....[They] started to realize that we're just human beings like everyone else, I guess.[30]

A new hospital building was transported by barge to Alert Bay and placed behind the old hospital, which was converted to a nurse's residence. The St. George's Hospital Society, made up of representatives of local White communities, took over the administration of the hospital from the Columbia Coast Mission in 1947, and in so doing brought in several changes to the hospital's policies. Recalling some of the difficulties involved in this transition, Historian Doris Andersen notes that during the days of mission administration,

> ...allowances were made...for Indian families to visit patients at all hours, respecting the Indian patients' desire to have family nearby during illness. Thus the *Columbia* would often bring in a boatload of relatives and their belongings as well as an Indian patient from some remote village. Other relatives in Alert Bay took in the visitors, and the patient, relaxed and reassured, was surrounded by familiar faces. The hospital informality during the years of mission administration was something the Indians missed when the government took over and strict regulations were enforced.[31]

From the beginning, two full-time, permanent doctors have been essential for the adequate running of the hospital. During the post-war years, Doris Andersen continues, "St. George's Hospital in Alert Bay was desperate, making do with a succession of relief doctors who changed at frequent intervals..."[32]

It was around this time, 1949 to be exact, that Dr. Harold J. "Jack" Pickup arrived and set up a permanent practice in Alert Bay. Based at St. George's, he made a name for himself during the early years as a "flying doctor," piloting his own plane around to the isolated logging camps and Indian villages he served.

The July, 1953 issue of the B.C. Hospital Insurance Service newsletter devoted a double page centre spread to Dr. Pickup:

> Standing on the beach 50 feet in front of the hospital, the administrator and the nurse anxiously watched the seaplane as it landed. Seconds later they were helping the pilot to carry the patient to the hospital. The 2000 inhabitants of Alert Bay heaved a sigh of relief. Their fabulous and youthful flying doctor, Dr. Jack Pickup, was home safely once again with one more mercy trip to add to the record in his log book.
>
> Thousands of loggers and fishermen, living on innumerable islands, inlets and lakes on the Northern part of Vancouver Island, in the Queen Charlotte and Johnston Straits and on the west coast of the mainland, owe their lives and limbs to the foresight and courage of the intrepid pilot-doctor.

Dr. Pickup invested in the burgeoning businesses of the area and his financial position was further enhanced by the advent of medicare in the 1960s. He became a leading local political figure, serving over the years as mayor, president of the Lions Club, and member of the Board of Trade. He soon became a shining symbol of the kind of humanitarian-pioneer so many of his colleagues saw themselves as. As interest in Indian health issues grew, Dr. Pickup was frequently called upon to serve on regional and province-wide committees concerned with this field, in which he came to be considered somewhat of an expert.

Tuberculosis and other respiratory ailments, particularly, still plagued the Native population, and the tradition begun in the 1900s of Indians donating money to support St. George's Hospital had continued. The hospital was desegregated, and in 1953, in keeping with the changing times, the Board of Trustees created a position for an Indian representative to sit on the annual fund-raising committee. The man chosen for this position was a hereditary chief, a successful fisherman, a devout Anglican, and a leading member of the Native Brotherhood of B.C. In his autobiography, James Sewid describes the occasion of his appointment:

For some years the white people in Alert Bay had formed a committee each year which tried to raise money to help support the hospital...I was the only Indian on the committee and they elected me to be the chairman of that committee, which was the first time that an Indian had been the chairman...Mr. Cameron, a friend of mine who was the Fisheries Officer, used to watch me like an old watchdog to see if I did anything as the chairman that wasn't according to parliamentary procedures.[33]

In 1947 British Columbia granted Indians the vote in provincial elections and the first Native M.L.A., Nis'ga Frank Calder, was elected to the legislature in Victoria in 1949. Revisions made to the Indian Act in 1951 dropped—but never repealed—the sections forbidding potlatching and the raising of money to support land claims organizing. The 1951 revisions also made it legal for Indians to drink in licensed premises but not to purchase, possess or drink alcohol anywhere else. Indian Agents began to be joined, and eventually replaced, by locally-elected Band Councils who remained, however, dependent upon, funded by, and accountable to, the Department of Indian Affairs. The Native Brotherhood officially expanded its mandate to include agitating for the settlement of land claims.

Alcohol had been prohibited to Indians by the Indian Act since 1876, and had had the effect, as had prohibition elsewhere, of driving the activity underground and criminalizing drinkers. At the same time, it created highly profitable possibilities for ambitious entrepreneurs. Of course, selling liquor to Indians had been lucrative since the early days of the fur trade, but the relatively high wages made by many Native men in the fishing industry made the late 1940s and '50s a boom time for bootleggers. Not a few young men came to the Kwakwaka'wakw area as penniless loggers, or greenhorn fishermen, and were able to sufficiently supplement their incomes by bootlegging liquor to Indians to enable them to open small businesses, or to purchase logging operations or fishing boats. Some became prominent members of their communities, taking their place alongside members of the already established "old" elite and participating in service clubs and organizations like the Royal Canadian Legion and the Lions Club.

Of course, not all white men were bootleggers. Nor, for that matter, were all bootleggers white men. Connections made through work, and the increasing number of inter-marriages, engendered a good deal of social interaction between white fishermen and loggers and the Native people of the Alert Bay region. Some suppliers of liquor were simply friends, in-laws, workmates— or Indians themselves who could "pass"— who purchased liquor for shared social occasions like week-end parties and weddings at no profit, and sometimes at risk, to themselves. But the incidence of alcohol-related deaths, particularly among young Native men, and incarceration for liquor offences under the terms of the Indian Act, increased significantly during this period.[34]

In 1960 the federal franchise was extended to Indians and all prohibitions concerning the purchase and consumption of alcohol were lifted. Local bootleggers suffered a setback when a provincial government liquor store was opened up in Alert Bay that same year. Continued prosperity from logging and fishing allowed Cormorant Island residents to own approximately 132 private cars and trucks[35] and the addition of a fleet of ten taxis and an ambulance travelling the island's four miles of paved road earned Alert Bay the distinction of appearing in the *Guinness Book of World Records* under the classification "Most Cars Per Mile of Road."

Potlatching came out in public again and during the 1960s Kwakwaka'wakw Big Houses were rebuilt in Victoria, Campbell River and Alert Bay. After sixty-seven years of legal injunction, the form and content of potlatch dances, songs and ritual appeared to have been only minimally modified.

Almost a century had gone by since the first missionaries and Indian Agents had pontificated in their journals and reports about the impending disappearance of the "inferior" races they had determined to civilize. Not only had previous government policies aimed at assimilation failed in their objectives, but almost 100 years after the Indian Act was first legislated, distinct Native communities continued to exist; the potlatch was undergoing a rejuvenation; the Kwakwala language, while no longer the mother tongue of most Alert Bay Indians, was still spoken by the old people and, given the persistence of the extended family, was at least partially understood by many of the young. An unprecedented "baby boom" had taken place during the 1950s and '60s and reserve populations across Canada mushroomed. By the end of the 1960s, tuberculosis had been brought under control and infant mortality rates were beginning to come down. Although alcohol-related accidents and diseases had replaced T.B. as the main health problem and cause of death, particularly among adults aged 20-40, in sheer numbers, the Native population promised to double in less than twenty years, and Indians were still organizing themselves politically to pursue a settlement of land claims.

Despite all these changes, the essential economic and political structure of Alert Bay remained relatively stable. An ethnographer working in one of the outlying villages in the mid-1960s, described Alert Bay as follows:

> The "white end" has a fleet of radio-dispatched taxis, two hotels with beer parlours, several stores, a bank, post office, government liquor store, a land and water detachment of the R.C.M.P., a hospital with three resident doctors, four cafes, local offices of three major fishing companies, several boat refueling stations, a volunteer fire department, several Protestant churches and resident ministers, a Canadian Legion clubhouse, two community halls, two movies, offices of the Department of Transport, the Department of Forestry, and the

Fish and Game Commission, and an elementary-high school which takes all local Indian and White children.

Alert Bay is a modern frontier town. As well as its permanent population the town is peopled by itinerant loggers and fishermen during parts of the year, men who occasionally bring money but who have no responsibilities in the town. It is also peopled by some minority groups, including a few Chinese merchants; a group of Europeans, primarily fishermen, referred to as "the Yugoslavs" or "D.P.'s"; a smattering of immigrants from all over the world; a few Americans; and some young people from bigger cities like Vancouver who hope to make high wages before returning home. The "elite" whites of Alert Bay keep their houses, their drinking habits, their social intercourse, and sometimes even their courtesy, to themselves.

Alert Bay is headquarters of the Kwawkewlth Indian Agency, staffed by an Agency Superintendent, an Assistant Superintendent, and an office staff of three. There is an Anglican residency for about 150 elementary school age Indian children who are brought in from outlying villages along the coast. In adjacent quarters is a clinic and residence for two nurses employed by the Indian Health Service.[36]

"The Village," or the "Indian End," remained strictly residential.

A renewed interest was taken in Indian education. The residential school system had failed to produce the expected results, and the philosophy of racialist paternalism upon which it was based had now become an embarrassing anachronism. A new approach to assimilation, more in keeping with the principles of a modern pluralist democracy, began to gain prominence. Beginning in 1955, Alert Bay Indians moved from the Indian Day School they had been attending to an integrated public school which was located on the White End, although it was generously financed by the Department of Indian Affairs. Children from the outlying villages continued to live at St. Mike's but began to attend public school as well.

While federally-funded residential schools were being closed down in favour of public day schools during the 1960s, the rate of apprehension of Native children by provincial social welfare authorities in British Columbia was increasing proportionately. In 1955 the number of Native children listed as wards of the provincial child welfare department in B.C. was almost nil. By 1964, Native children comprised one-third of all children "in care." Institutionalization of Native children away from their own families and communities had moved from federal to provincial jurisdiction.[37] Patrick Johnson, in his book *Native Children and the Child Welfare System*, documents the rationale underlying this approach:

One longtime employee of the Ministry of Human Resources in B.C....admitted that provincial social workers would, quite literally,

90

scoop children from reserves on the slightest pretext. She also made it clear, however, that she and her colleagues sincerely believed that what they were doing was in the best interests of the children. They felt that the apprehension of Indian children from reserves would save them from the effects of crushing poverty, unsanitary health conditions, poor housing and malnutrition, which were facts of life on many reserves. Unfortunately, the long-term effect of apprehension on the individual child was not considered. More likely, it could not have been imagined. Nor were the effects of apprehension on Indian families and communities taken in account and some reserves lost almost a generation of their children as a result.[38]

The velvet glove still concealed an iron fist.

In 1970, Alan Fry, Indian Agent for the Kwakiutl District during the 1960s, published a novel, *How A People Die*, which was set in an unnamed, modern Indian village. While the western world had, for the most part, rejected the kind of crude evolutionism which had characterized the thinking of nineteenth-century colonists, Fry found it appropriate to describe the thoughts and feelings of a contemporary, fictional, local doctor as he reflected on his practice among Indians in terms which William Halliday would likely have found agreeable:

> The trouble, Dr. Cooper thought, was that the simple maxims of survival no longer apply.
>
> Before all the paraphernalia of the modern society—medical science with its phalanx of technology and equipment and doctors and nurses, social welfare agencies to parcel out subsistence and apprehend the victims of neglect, preventive immunology to limit the ravage of disease, government housing to house those who would never have housed themselves—before all that the children of the ineffectual parents survived in such few numbers.
>
> In an animal species living directly in the natural environment, those faulty by the standards of the species will fail to survive long enough to reproduce in any quantity. In the same way it had always come about that the slovenly people, unable to function effectively in the social and economic environment of man's less advanced communities, would bring only a few of their children to survive into adulthood....
>
> The dynamics of this process are not kind. They serve the race, not the individual. Nature tolerates with equanimity the perishing of some and the surviving of others.
>
> But now modern man has decided to defy nature. He has said that everyone to whom life has been given by the persistent capacity of man to reproduce shall have the use of some space, the opportunity to live, the opportunity to reproduce...

Not only the fit survive. So also do the unfit.

It is so very decent. Dr. Cooper, whose knowledge and skills were devoted to restoring and preserving life began to wonder if, ultimately, it was workable.[39]

"The times they are a'changin'," went the lyrics of a popular song of the day, and indeed they were. But Native peoples must be forgiven if they appear to maintain a certain degree of scepticism about just how much and how fast times really do change.

V. BUT NOT ANY MORE (?) ....THE '70s

DECLARATION OF SOVEREIGNTY
THAT the Nimpkish River, Nimpkish Lake and estuaries are now and have always been the exclusive property of the Nimpkish Indian Band.

THAT the preservation of these waters in their natural state is essential to the survival of the Nimpkish people and other native peoples of this area.

THAT in order to guarantee that these resources are preserved a freeze be placed on all development, sale or lease of all private and government land in the area, all industrial activities, camping, and any activity which may now or in future affect these waters in any way.

THAT this freeze remain in effect until such time as a just and equitable settlement is made of both the general land claim of the Nimpkish Indian Band and the interim claim of the river, lake and estuaries being made now.

—Nimpkish Band Council, November, 1975

1969 was another major turning point for Canadian Indians. It was in this year that newly-elected Prime Minister Pierre Trudeau published his now infamous "White Paper Policy." The essential thrust of the White Paper Policy was that reserves be converted into municipalities, the Indian Act be repealed, "Indian status" done away with entirely, and Native people integrated-assimilated into mainstream Canadian society as quickly as possible. While the government claimed that "this policy rests upon the fundamental right of Indian people to full and equal participation in the cultural, social, economic and political life of Canada,"[40] Indian leaders across the country interpreted the motives behind the White Paper quite differently. To them, there was little if anything "new" about it.

Native representatives had participated in a series of consultations with the federal government prior to the publication of the policy where they had made it very clear that they considered the settlement of long outstanding grievances regarding land rights and self-determination to be their first priority. The resulting

White Paper, however, denied recognition of aboriginal title, or land claims, as a basis for negotiating a new relationship between Indians and the Canadian state, and was thoroughly assimilationist in its philosophy and program. One Native leader expressed the general feeling among Canadian Indians following the announcement of this new (old) policy when he said: "I feel like a man who has been told he must die and am now to be consulted on the method of implementing the decision."[41]

Given this negative response on the part of Native leaders, the federal government officially withdrew the White Paper Policy and chose instead to create and fund provincial and national Native organizations who were mandated to conduct land claims research in order that Natives could better prepare for the long-awaited negotiation of a land claim settlement, which everyone now assumed was imminent. The 1970s were therefore a decade of unprecedented public militancy on the part of Indians all over Canada, and Alert Bay soon became known as one of the more vocal hotbeds of this militancy in British Columbia.

When federal government funding was made available to support social and economic development projects like small businesses on the reserve, local government infrastructures for bands, and reserve-based social services, the non-Indian community became increasingly defensive of their economic security, and of the relatively privileged social positions they had held for so long. Naturally, these developments meant that during the '70s the relationship beween the Native and non-Native communities in Alert Bay was particularly strained.

When an Indian Fisherman's Assistance Program (IFAP) aimed at guaranteeing an on-going Indian presence in the commercial fishery was instituted, despite the fact that Indian participation in the industry had been declining dramatically, IFAP was seen by many non-Indian fishermen, also struggling to survive in a flagging industry, as giving Indians an unfair advantage. Not only did a few Native fishermen get big, new boats, but the Native Brotherhood renewed its agitation for special harvesting rights for aboriginal fishermen. Tensions therefore increased between Alert Bay's Native Brotherhood local, which represented most of the Native fishermen, and the United Fishermen's and Allied Workers Union to which the town's non-Native fishermen belonged.

A food co-op was organized on the reserve which, for a while at least, reduced the take in the local grocery stores. A revolt against the public school began, and culminated in the establishment of an independent, band-administered school. When the Nimpkish Band Council declared sovereignty over the entire Nimpkish Valley, an active Land Claims Committee enforced it by means of public demonstrations, including the closing of a bridge and the exacting of a toll to enter Indian Land.

The fishing and logging industries upon which the region depended slid more deeply into recession during the 1970s and the new Island Highway made transportation by water an anachronism. Alert Bay's historical position as the centre of the region declined proportionately as towns on the mainland and along the Island Highway grew. The municipality's Board of Trade commissioned local Native artists to carve a 180-foot totem pole, which they raised in front of the Big House, and Alert Bay made it into the *Guinness Book of World Records* once again, as it now boasted "The World's Tallest Totem Pole."

While the non-Indian businessmen pinned their hopes for "economic renewal" on establishing a tourist mecca, the Land Claims Committee posted a large billboard decorated with a majestic killer whale's face at the ferry dock. An arrow on the bottom of the sign pointed left—to the Village—and read NIMPKISH INDIAN LAND, while another arrow, pointing right—to the White End—declared STOLEN NIMPKISH INDIAN LAND.[42]

These challenges, of course, often generated much anger and resentment within the non-Indian community. There were those, however, who, like the man who served as mayor of the municipality from 1974 onward, tried to bridge the gulf and encourage everyone to work together for the greater good of the whole town. When journalists interviewed Mayor Popovich about racial tensions in Alert Bay in 1979, their report read as follows:

> When told that some Indians talk angrily of opening their own stores so they won't have to deal with white merchants, Mayor Popovich sighed and said: 'The Indians are becoming more self-reliant and I cannot blame them for that. They want to form their own cooperatives and create employment, better standards of living...it's long overdue...their rights...'[43]

However, despite the many confrontations, conferences, programs and projects which characterized reserve life during the 1970s, fundamentally, little changed. The basic social and economic structure of Alert Bay was, by 1979, still essentially the same as it had been for over 100 years.

The Indian community consisted of the Nimpkish Indian Reserve with a population of about 1000, and the Whe-La-La-U All-Bands Reserve where about 150 members of Kwakwaka'wakw bands other than the Nimpkish lived. Social status continued to be determined by a complex web of relationships in which status was defined partly by individual achievement and partly by family affiliation, partly by the potlatch hierarchy and partly by the degree of success obtained in contemporary economic and political structures. In this latter category there were the few seine boat owners; a few more who were skippers of seine boats owned by fishing companies; men who were steadily employed as crews on fishing boats; Band Councillors, most of whom were either boat owners or skippers, and band administration staff and other band employees, mostly women who were involved in social service work. Native women also worked as cooks on fishboats, as waitresses, taxi drivers, and as kitchen and maintenance staff at the hospital. The remainder of the Indian population, approximately half, were fairly steadily unemployed and therefore depended on social assistance for their livelihood. In recent years, with the decline of the fishing industry and increased funding of local administration, the two most rapidly growing sectors of the reserve community were band employees and welfare recipients. Everyone, to varying extents, relied upon subsistence activities to supplement their diet.

On the reserve in 1979 there was a small band school, a cafeteria, a liquor lounge, band administration offices, and a variety of economic development projects, none of which had been around long enough to be considered stable features of the community. There were no stores on the reserve, with the exception of a few "bread and candy" operations some women ran from their homes.

The traditional potlatch hierarchy spanned all categories of the contemporary one, and family ties crossed status lines. To be successful in contemporary terms, and to have maintained a high rank within the potlatch system, as, for example, the Dicks and some others had done, located a family at the top of both scales, and placed them unequivocally in what could be called the "Indian elite." Conversely, to have neither succeeded in the new context, nor to have kept up obligations in the old, placed a family at the bottom of both scales. Most, naturally, fell somewhere in between.

The population of the White End consisted of permanent residents and transients. Permanent residents included both descendants of the early pioneer homesteaders, administrators and entrepreneurs, and people who had settled in town at various times since the 1920s. Most, however, had arrived during the post-war boom years of the late 1940s and '50s. Transients were people who came to town to work for relatively short periods of time, not intending to stay.

The majority of the permanent population was made up of families of fishermen and loggers, workers-turned-small-businessmen, and tradesmen, the women of which were sometimes clerical workers in the stores, the hospital, the banks, and in fishing company and government offices. Some worked as cooks on fishboats, as nurses and as taxi drivers. People from this sector comprised the membership of community organizations and service clubs. Many had inter-married with Native families, often the men were fishermen, and since 1955 young people from both communities who grew up in Alert Bay attended the same schools and socialized together as a matter of course. Also included in this sector were former transients such as teachers and nurses who had either married into Alert Bay families or who had settled permanently in town.

Fishing, telephone and hydro company employees, nurses, teachers, R.C.M.P. officers, hospital technical staff, bank employees, and other government workers made up the transient sector. While some permanent residents were employed in such capacities, most of these positions were filled by people putting in time awaiting promotion and transfer to a more urban locale. These people saved their money, took their vacations away, and while in town associated almost entirely with the White community, often socializing privately among themselves rather than going out to the bars, and dealing with Indians only in their official capacities. Since this group most often consisted of single people or young couples with no children or very young children, they tended not to become involved in matters of local concern, such as education and health care, which bring people with families together in such communities.

There was also a small Oriental group, most of whom had lived in town since the 1940s. Their three small stores were located in close proximity to each other on a strip of road nick-named "Chinatown." "Chinatown" is about an eighth of a mile south of the main cluster of White-owned stores, which is referred to as "Downtown." While none of these families were tightly integrated into either community, their social and business associations were primarily with the White community.

During the '60s and '70s, dope dealers and American draft dodgers joined itinerant loggers, fishermen, bootleggers, artists and eccentrics in the ever present, but always changing, population of people considered "strangers" by both Indians and Whites.

As well as permanent residents and transients, the non-Indian population could also be hierarchically grouped in categories based on occupational status. Of course, in a small community the social boundaries of such categories tend to be more blurred than in an urban situation. A single family may include individuals from each occupational category, and people from all groups may belong to the same community, religious and service clubs, and hence socialize together and inter-marry frequently. Nevertheless, an identifiable "White elite" which was particularly influential in shaping understandings of local history, politics, and relations with Indians, was prominent.

At the top of Alert Bay's non-Native hierarchy in 1979, were, as ever, families of the long-established and prosperous businessmen, the doctor, the coroner, the hospital and school administrative staff, the R.C.M.P. Sergeant, and elderly people now retired from similar positions. This elite included permanent residents who were descendants of the original settler families as well as more recent arrivals, and a few transients like the high school principal and his wife. Permanent residents of long standing however, were the most influential members. Although some had lived in town for generations, for the most part their children had been sent away to private schools, and encouraged to settle elsewhere. Members of this elite were active in local politics and were the leaders of community and service clubs. Women in this sector were often particularly active volunteers in organizations like the St. George's Hospital Ladies' Auxiliary and the Alert Bay Library and Museum. Their social standing, their backgrounds, and their long experience in the region gave them a significant degree of prestige and they were looked up to within their community. Dr.

Pickup was a leading member of this elite, having been mayor for many years before being replaced by Gilbert Popovitch in 1974. In 1979, Dr. Pickup was president of the Royal Canadian Legion and the Board of Trade.

The White elite was firmly entrenched, both economically and ideologically, in the historical structure of the town, and their relationships with the Native community continued to be played out in two main forums: private businesses; and public institutions for the medical care, education and policing—or caretaking—of the Indian community. Economically, maintenance of the local status quo required that Indians remain dependent and passive consumers of products and services. One Native woman described this relationship as it persisted in 1979: "They may not like us," she explained, "but they need our money. And we need their stores." Ideologically, this status quo relied on Indians being thought of as incapable of meeting their own needs, and as being grateful for their caretakers. The contradiction which may seem obvious to some—that is, that the relative prosperity and social prestige enjoyed by this sector of the White community depended on the corresponding want and dependency of the Indian community—does not figure in this way of thinking which remains rooted in the principles of nineteenth-century philanthropy.

Of all the institutions that existed in Alert Bay in 1979, the one that most exemplified, personified and perpetuated the historical, colonial structure of Alert Bay society, and the relationships which are supported by such a base, was St. George's Hospital. Not only did professional and semi-professional employment at the hospital provide a relatively good income in the context of Alert Bay, but it also maintained a social relationship which, like that between the businessmen and the Indian community, was as old as the town itself.

The St. George's Hospital Society Board of Trustees consisted of eleven members.[44] Two were appointed: one by the Lieutenant-Governor and one by the Board of the Regional Hospital District. In 1978-79 these positions were held by two members of Alert Bay's white elite. The other nine Trustees were elected by the St. George's Hospital Society to represent the communities served by the hospital. These positions were divided up as follows: three representatives from the Municipality of Alert Bay; one each from the four Vancouver Island communities of Beaver Cove, Telegraph Cove, Port McNeill and the District of Port Hardy; one from neighbouring Sointula on Malcolm Island and one from each of the Kwakwaka'wakw communities. The Society's Constitution and By-Laws allowed for the various communities to be represented by non-residents if necessary. The Chairman of the Hospital Board at the time of Renee Smith's death was Sointula's representative, a Pentecostal clergyman. The Vice-Chairperson was one of the Municipality of Alert Bay's representatives, an ex-nurse, long-time permanent resident and member of the white elite, now employed by the provincial Ministry of Human Resources. The other two representatives of the White End were the high school principal's wife and the wife of a prominent local businessman. Coroner Deadman, of Alert

ST. GEORGE'S HOSPITAL*

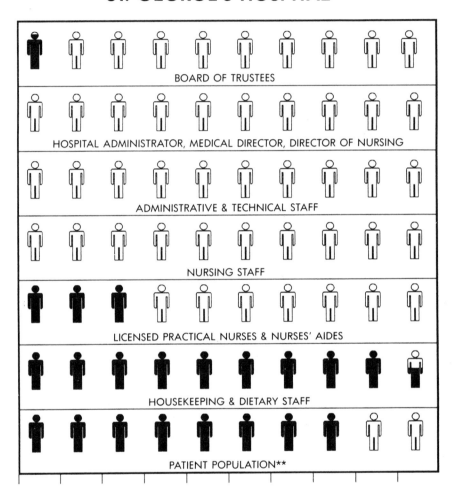

BOARD OF TRUSTEES

HOSPITAL ADMINISTRATOR, MEDICAL DIRECTOR, DIRECTOR OF NURSING

ADMINISTRATIVE & TECHNICAL STAFF

NURSING STAFF

LICENSED PRACTICAL NURSES & NURSES' AIDES

HOUSEKEEPING & DIETARY STAFF

PATIENT POPULATION**

*proportions based on composition at 1979–80

**includes both status and non-status Indians (50–80%)

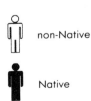

non-Native

Native

98

Bay, served as the representative of the District of Port Hardy. Beaver Cove and Telegraph Cove were represented by members of those communities and Port McNeill was represented by a member of the Nimpkish Band who had become a successful logging contractor and who no longer lived on reserve. Another member of the Nimpkish Band, resident on the reserve in Alert Bay and a long-standing supporter of the hospital, represented all the Kwakwaka'wakw communities. Of the eleven positions on the hospital's Board of Trustees, therefore, six were held by members of Alert Bay's white elite, two by members of the Nimpkish Band (one of whom represented the non-Indian community of Port McNeill) and three were held by residents of other local non-Indian communities.

St. George's staff was jointly headed by a Medical Director, Dr. Pickup, and a British-born administrator who was a permanent resident of long standing. The Nursing Director was also British and the Head Nurse was a Euro-Canadian woman who had married into one of the old settler families on the island. There was a large turnover in the few Registered Nurse positions and these tended to be filled by young, non-Native women, often wives of transient government functionaries putting in their time in Alert Bay. Most of the duties usually carried out by R.N.s in larger centres were performed at St. George's by Graduate Nurses from the Philippines. These women had graduated from R.N. training programs in their home country but had not obtained Canadian certification. Frequently, they were recent immigrants who worked in rural hospitals like St. George's hoping to improve their command of English and to gain the experience necessary to upgrade their qualifications and eventually move on. The lab technicians were both Euro-Canadians and Filipino-Canadians, as were most of the Licensed Practical Nurses (L.P.N.s) and Nurses' Aides. 20 per cent of the hospital staff were Native women, employed in the kitchen and the maintenance departments. Indians made up 50-80 per cent of the hospital's patients. Most were admitted for alcohol-related problems.

While health care workers and professionals obviously provide needed services and do valuable work, there is a tendency for their social status—and sometimes their sense of personal identity—to rely on the assumption that qualifications in the health care field not only indicate the successful completion of specialized training, but also confer a certain degree of moral superiority upon those who obtain them. This attitude can become even more exaggerated among those who deal primarily with patients who suffer from socially-stigmatized diseases like alcoholism. In the context of a community like Alert Bay, where health care personnel are non-Indian, and patients are Indian, assumptions of cultural or racial superiority intensify individual self-righteousness and professional snobbery and most often add an element of paternalism to the relationship between professionals and patients. Among transient health care personnel, if these attitudes existed, they were further exacerbated by the fact that while health care personnel worked for members of the White elite who ran the hospital, and socialized primarily with non-Natives and other transients, they often encountered Native people only as patients.

Such structures and ways of thinking insulate health care personnel, and other caretakers, against criticism from Native people, and encourage the perpetuation of a double standard when comparing Indians and Whites, which is held so uncritically that it comes to be seen as common sense. While lamenting the inferiority of Indian people and, particularly, some of their life-styles, caretakers simultaneously reinforce notions of their own superiority. Were an observer to suggest that, often in the areas of drinking and sexual liaisons, the differences are more ones of style than of actual participation in the activity, one would find few in this group who would agree. There were, and are, of course, always a minority of individuals to whom these descriptions do not apply, but they tended to be the exceptions who proved the rule.

In 1979, St. George's Hospital's existence was being challenged by developments both inside and outside the community of Alert Bay. Since the early 1970s discussions had been taking place among municipal, regional and provincial authorities as to how best to allocate health care resources in the North Island district. Arguments for drastically reducing the size and functions of St. George's were many and convincing. With new, more modern and better-equipped hospitals being built in nearby towns on Vancouver Island connected by the new highway, and with Air-Sea Rescue ambulances able to take patients from Alert Bay to hospitals in Vancouver and Victoria in little more time than it takes to drive across a city in an ambulance, it was argued that Alert Bay now only required an emergency facility with a few beds. In defending the need to maintain a fully-equipped—and, more importantly, fully-staffed—facility in Alert Bay, hospital and municipal representatives relied upon statistics and "expert professional opinions" which claimed that the Indian population being served by St. George's possessed distinctive characteristics that led them to require and use hospital facilities to a greater extent than a non-Indian population of the same size.

In 1974, the British Columbia Medical Association (BCMA)'s Federal/Provincial Committee on Indian Health—to which Dr. Pickup was appointed a corresponding member—published a report whose findings supported the rationale being put forward by St. George's in the battle to maintain the size of the hospital. The Committee's main findings, under the heading INDIAN HEALTH PROBLEMS AND ATTITUDES, were as follows:

In comparison to most non-Indians, Indians often
(a) fail to recognize early symptoms of illness;
(b) have a higher tolerance for pain and discomfort and a fatalistic acceptance of things as they are;
(c) present [themselves] in the acute and often fatal stages of an illness.

Complications in treatment occur because many Indians have multiple ailments and also because their general health is poor and follow-up treatment is accepted only reluctantly if at all.

In a few instances, medical treatment is delayed until traditional treatment has been explored often causing serious delays in the instigation of necessary medical treatment.

It is the impression of the Committee...that Indian patients tend to remain in hospital for longer periods of time because of the frequent presence of inter-allied disorders and because of the many difficulties often associated with the adequate provision of nursing or boarding home facilities, transportation, and also adequate medical follow-up....The pattern of not following medical instructions adequately and not returning for follow-up care is an important consideration in the treatment of Indian patients. The lack of concern for follow-up care is one of the factors contributing not only to the frequent hospitalization of patients but also to a longer hospital stay.

In 1974 the Regional District of Mount Waddington, whose jurisdiction included Alert Bay, Sointula, Port McNeill, Port Alice and Port Hardy, voted to build one central district hospital on Vancouver Island and emergency units in the smaller towns. Alert Bay's distinctive situation was acknowledged in that towns with comparable population numbers were given three-bed to ten-bed units while St. George's received a modern X-ray unit, a new laboratory and its total official capacity remained at fifty-five beds. In a report to the Municipal Council, however, Dr. Pickup cautioned that despite these improvements, if plans for the new district hospital went ahead, St. George's would inevitably be reduced to a ten-bed emergency clinic. In his report Dr. Pickup stated:

The whole question comes down to a matter of philosophy. Is it better to have doctors and hospitals at Port Alice, Port Hardy, Port McNeill and Alert Bay, or at Port McNeill only? There are plenty of arguments on both sides. Personally I believe that better overall medical care can be given by having the doctors where the people are and sufficient beds in the various centers to care for the 80%-90% of cases that can be dealt with locally.[45]

Nevertheless, it was a losing battle. Complaints about Dr. Pickup, easier access to doctors in larger centres, and the general trend toward medical specialization had, for several years, prompted the more affluent and more mobile members of the local Indian and non-Indian communities to seek medical care outside Alert Bay whenever possible. St. George's, and Dr. Pickup, had thus come increasingly to rely on a patient population which consisted primarily of Indians from the outlying villages, many of whom conformed to the stereotypical images held of them by many medical professionals. This group constituted a "captive clientele" for the hospital. Other regular patients were townspeople who did not, for one reason or another, leave the island very often; chronic alcoholics—Indian and non-Indian—from the whole region; and people loyal to either Dr. Pickup or St. George's, or both. Everyone in Alert Bay, of course, relied upon Dr. Pickup and St. George's for emergency care; but, for the most part, people who could, or who thought they could, sought attention elsewhere for serious medical problems.

Despite all the turmoil going on in town following Renee Smith's death, the hospital administrator wrote the following letter, on February 28, 1979, to the Nimpkish Band Council, requesting their co-operation in keeping St. George's open:

> Dear Mrs. Alfred, Band Manager:
> At a recent meeting of the Mount Waddington Regional Hospital Committee suggestions were made that when a new hospital facility is erected in Port Hardy, St. George's may be reduced to a ten-bed hospital...
> As approximately 50% of St. George's Hospital patients are from the Native people, we urgently seek your support in anyway possible, to retain at least 25 beds in Alert Bay....[46]

The Band Council replied on March 7, 1979:

> We agree that 10 beds would be inadequate but at this time we would like to know what the board's position is regarding the current controversy centering around Dr. Pick-up and his drinking problem. There is a very definite increase in the number of people, Indian and non-Indian, who are travelling to Vancouver Island or the mainland to seek medical attention and this surely will be reflected in records of the hospital use. We would like to know how the board will be dealing with this issue.[47]

The Hospital Board responded promptly on March 9, 1979:

> It goes without saying, that the Board of Trustees are extremely concerned about the quality of medical care and services provided to the people of both Cormorant Island and the surrounding localities, and have spent many long hours towards this goal.
> The amount of monies spent in providing services to this hospital for the comfort and benefit of the population at large has indeed been heavy as no doubt you may have observed by the many improvements that we have made towards the quality of care.

Regarding your inquiry into the habits of our local physician, every effort has been made by my board to arrive at a fair and judicious conclusion, having the interest at heart of every member of the community. We ask that you place your trust in our board and support us in our endeavours.[48]

Therefore, in the furor caused by Renee's death, the petitions, and the accusations made by the Public Health Nurse in her radio broadcast, the stakes were high for all concerned. Not only was there the immediate fear that the hospital would be closed down, or its services and staffing requirements severely curtailed, but also the moral and ideological underpinnings of a 100-year-old relationship between an indigenous community and a settler population were being challenged at their very core.

For many local people, therefore, the choice of what position to take regarding the controversy was anything but simple and straightforward and within the Indian community there was not unanimity. Everyone had something to fear in taking up a fight such as this one.

Some of the Indian women who worked in the hospital's kitchen and maintenance departments feared losing their jobs and found the daily pressure and antagonism they received from their supervisors since this scandal had erupted too hard to bear.

Others, like Renee's mother, Margaret, went to work each day, avoided arguments and stuck to their guns.

Many people respected Dr. Pickup for what he had been and felt personally indebted to him for saving their lives, or the life of someone close to them.

Some had never seen another doctor.

Some sincerely judged him to be a competent doctor.

Others feared losing their credit at the local stores owned by Dr. Pickup's supporters.

Still others feared being cut off their easy, ever-renewable prescriptions and regular sojourns in the hospital.

Some did not want to "cause trouble" and said starting a fight would only make things worse because "Indians always lose."

Some wished to avoid arguments with other members of their families, their non-Indian in-laws, or both.

Some didn't like the Dick family or the Band Council and were reluctant to support anything they did.

Everyone feared themselves or their children getting sick in the middle of the night and having to turn to Dr. Pickup for help after publicly criticizing him.

No one wanted to lose the hospital.

Many of the elderly Indian people also defended Dr. Pickup, although, as time went on, they often saw other doctors at their children's insistence. These

"Old People" had desperately needed medical care for themselves and their families for most of their lives, and had not always received what they required. They had long ago deferred to medical authority; and doctors, missionaries, administrators, and businessmen had formed the ruling cliques under which they had lived most of their lives. Their loyalty to the doctor, and their reluctance to publicly criticize authorities, was rooted in a lifetime of experiences with which many of the younger people were sympathetic, but impatient. Whereas young people made cracks about "ol' Doc Kill'em'quick," their parents and grandparents remembered incidents in the villages, or on the fishing grounds, or in logging camps, when someone had been clinging precariously to life after a serious illness or accident and Dr. Pickup had appeared and saved the day. Women defended their support of the doctor by saying, "That man delivered all my children! And my grandchildren!" Others thought the doctor should be asked to resign, but quietly and politely.

For still others, particularly those of us who worked in community development and band administration, or who were on the Band Council, it seemed contradictory to be, on the one hand, fighting for the settlement of land claims and for greater economic and educational opportunities, while, at the same time, allowing the local doctor and hospital to go on giving Indians such poor care. In our eyes, the relationship between Native people and Dr. Pickup and St. George's epitomized, on the local level, the archaic colonial dependency we had committed ourselves to bringing to an end.

Regardless of all these complicating factors, however, a majority of people in the Village signed the petitions because "everyone knew it was all true," and the Band and District Councils stood firm.

"Going down the road" is what just about everyone on the reserve does just about every day. Going down the road means going to the business section of the White End, located in the centre of the island, about two miles from the northern-most point of the reserve. To shop, bank, collect mail, have a beer, buy a newspaper, visit someone in hospital, see a movie, go to school, it is necessary to go down the road. Down the road is where the formal transactions between the two communities are carried out and down the road is where one runs into everyone else from both the Village and the White End. It is virtually impossible to avoid going down the road or to predict whom one will be forced to interact with once there. As the positions became more polarized and consolidated into a Whites vs. Indians issue, going down the road became increasingly tense. Teachers complained that their classes were becoming unmanageable as children aligned themselves with their parents and families and carried the feud into the schools.

Everyone experienced at least some strain within their families and/or their jobs as a result of the controversy, and conflict within families in an Indian community is extremely painful. Not only are relationships multi-faceted, but they are also intense as daily life is lived in constant contact and social inter-action. In the complex web of relationships that bind people together in a town like Alert Bay, conflicting loyalties of the most personal, intimate and painful nature pulled members of both communities in several different directions. In the final analysis, however, the middle ground dissolved rapidly and only two sides emerged: Indian and White. By the time the Inquest opened on April 18, 1979, everyone had chosen sides. With few exceptions, Indians either sup-ported the "anti-Pickup" side or were silent. With few exceptions, Whites either supported the "pro-Pickup" side or were silent.

Silent or vocal, Indian or White, everyone placed their faith in the inquest to vindicate their positions.

NOTES:

[1]This a description written by non-Indians resident in the region and quoted in a book published by the 1958 Alert Bay Centennial Committee dedicated to the pioneers of the district. It was reprinted in 1971 as a British Columbia Centennial project.

This book, called *History of Alert Bay and District*, was compiled from published and unpublished memoirs written by the early non-Indian settlers in the Alert Bay area and supplemented by interviews with their descendants and successors. The book relies substantially on an account written by William Halliday in 1935, entitled *Potlatch and Totem: Memoirs of an Indian Agent*. Halliday is best known as having been a particularly fierce champion of colonial policy and was responsible for the prosecution of many Kwakwaka'wakw under the anti-potlatch law which came into effect in 1884. As well as being an Indian Agent for many years, Halliday was originally a homesteader, and later served as a lay missionary and school principal. Hence he was a very power-ful local figure. I use this particular book extensively as a reference source for descrip-tions of the permanent non-Indian communities' (particularly the sector I identify as the "white elite") interpretation of local history, and their understanding of their rela-tionship to the Kwakwaka'wakw, for several reasons. First, *History of Alert Bay and District* claims to be the settlers' story, told in their own words, and is still for sale in the town's drug store. Second, it is advertised and sold as a historically-accurate account. Third, to my knowledge, none of the people whose history and opinions it claims to represent have ever publicly voiced any objections to its content or to the manner in which they are represented by it. Finally, it is my opinion, and the opinion of many members of the Indian bands of the region, that, although the language used in this book is somewhat old-fashioned, it remains an accurate reflection of both the historical origins of the attitudes of some local non-Indians, particularly long time residents, towards Indians, and the contemporary persistence of these attitudes.

[2]Codere, Helen (ed) (1966) *Kwakiutl Ethnography: Franz Boas*, Chicago: Univer-sity of Chicago Press, pp. 361-362; 376-388.

[3]Billy Sandy Willie, Jack Peters, Jane Willie, Ethel Alfred, Agnes Alfred, Agnes Cranmer, Emma Beans, Bob Joseph and Gloria Cranmer Webster, presentation to *The Goldthorpe Inquiry*, (1980) Transcript: Vol. I, pp. 27-114.

[4]Codere, Helen (ed) (1966) *Kwakiutl Ethnography: Franz Boas*, Chicago: Univer-sity of Chicago Press, pp. 361-362; 376-388.

[5]Ibid., pp. 120-148.

[6]Ibid.

[7]Ibid.

[8]Vancouver, George (1798) *A Voyage of Discovery to the North Pacific Ocean, and Round the World;...Performed in the Years 1790, 1791, 1792, 1793, 1794, and 1795, in the "Discovery" Sloop of War, and Armed Tender "Chatham," under the Command of Captain George Vancouver*, London: G.G. and J. Robinson, Vol. 2, p. 292

[9]Wike, Joyce (1951) *Effect of the Maritime Fur Trade on Northwest Coast Indian Society*, Ph.D. dissertation, New York: Columbia University.

[10]Gloria Cranmer Webster, Wedledi Speck and Ernie Willie, presentations to *The Goldthorpe Inquiry,* (1980) Transcript: Vol. I, pp. 59-130.

[11]Duff, Wilson (1965) *The Indian History of British Columbia, Vol. 1: The Impact of the White Man*, Anthropology in British Columbia, Memoir No. 5, Victoria: Provincial Museum of British Columbia, p. 42, quoted in Gloria Cranmer Webster's presentation to *The Goldthorpe Inquiry,* (1980), Transcript: Vol. I, pp. 62-63.

[12]Collison, William Henry (1981) *In Wake of the War Canoe*, edited and annotated by Charles Lilliard, Victoria: Sono Nis Press, p. 68.

[13]Curtis, Edward (1905) *The North American Indian*, Vol. 10, New York: Johnson Reprint Company, p. 303.

Census data for this period of time is, of course, imprecise. Estimates for the size of the aboriginal Kwakwaka'wakw population range from 7000-12,000, placing Work's figures in the middle to high range of estimates. By all calculations, however, losses during the fifty years 1835-1885 hover between 70 per cent and 90 per cent for all the coastal aboriginal groups in British Columbia.

[14]Gloria Cranmer Webster and Wedledi Speck, presentations to: *The Goldthorpe Inquiry,* (1980) Transcript: Vol. 1, pp. 59-94.

[15]Halliday, William (1935) *Potlatch and Totem: Memoirs of an Indian Agent*, Toronto: J. M. Dent & Sons Ltd., pp. 226-227 and quoted in *History of Alert Bay and District*, op cit., p. 20, with the judicious omission of the disparaging description of the class origins of the white men.

[16]Foucault, Michel (1975) *The Birth of the Clinic*, New York: Random House, p. 42

[17]Lillard, Charles (ed) (1984) *Warriors of the North Pacific: Missionary Accounts of the Northwest Coast, the Skeena and Stikine Rivers and the Klondike 1829-1900*, Victoria: Sono Nis Press, p. 188.

[18]*History of Alert Bay and District*, op. cit., pp. 25-26.

[19]Tobias, John L. (1983) "Protection, Civilization, Assimilation: An Outline History of Canada's Indian Policy," in Getty, Ian A. L. and Antoine S. Lussier (eds), *As Long as the Sun Shines and Water Flows: A Reader in Canadian Native Studies*, Vancouver: University of British Columbia Press.

[20]McDonnell, C.E., M.D. (1978), "B.C. Medical History: Early Medical Legislation," *B. C. Medical Journal*, Vol. 20, No. 2, February p. 45

[21]Rose, Dr. T. F (1972) *From Shaman to Modern Medicine: A Century of the Healing Arts in British Columbia.* Vancouver: Mitchell Press Limited, p. 6.

[22]Ibid., p. 13.

[23]McKechnie, Robert E. II. M.D. (1972) *Strong Medicine: History of healing on the Northwest Coast*, Vancouver: J. J. Douglas, Ltd., p. 14.

[24]Sources for population data:

(a) B.C. Non-Indians: 1885 from Beaujot, R. and McQuillan, K. (1982) *Growth and Dualism*, Gage Publishing Ltd., p. 25; 1900-1980 from Province of British Columbia, Ministry of Health, Vital Statistics, *Annual Report*, 1980, p. 19.

(b) B.C. Indians: 1835-1954 from Hawthorne, H. (ed) (1966), *A Survey of the Contemporary Indians of Canada, Part 1*, Ottawa: Queen's Printer, p. 58; 1961 from Census Canada; 1980 from D.I.A.N.D. membership lists, Pacific Region.

(c) Kwakwa̲ka'wakw: Department of Indian Affairs records, researched by the writer during the summer of 1984. The figures represent the total membership of bands classified as part of the Kwakiutl Agency at various times and therefore represent slightly different groupings at different periods. General trends, however, can be accurately derived from these figures.

[25]Andersen, Doris (1982), *The Columbia Is Coming!*, Sidney, B.C.: Gray's Publishing Ltd., pp. 56-57.

[26]Gloria Cranmer Webster, presentation to *The Goldthorpe Inquiry*, (1980) Transcript: Vol. 1, p. 68.

[27]*History of Alert Bay and District*, op. cit. pp. 30-40.

[28]Ernest Willie, presentation to *The Goldthorpe Inquiry*, (1980) Transcript: Vol. 1, pp. 94-113.

[29]Jack Peters, presentation to *The Goldthorpe Inquiry*, (1980) Transcript: Vol. 1, p. 48

[30]Speck, George Jr., unpublished field notes, June 1983.

[31]Andersen, Doris (1982) *The Columbia is Coming!* op. cit., p. 57.

[32]Ibid., p. 180.

[33]Spradley, James (ed) (1969), *Guests Never Leave Hungry: The Autobiography of James Sewid, a Kwakiutl Indian*, Kingston: McGill-Queen's University Press, p. 158.

[34]Speck, George Jr., unpublished field notes.

[35]*History of Alert Bay and District*, op. cit., p. 94.

[36]Wolcott, H. F. (1964) *A Kwakiutl Village and Its School: Cultural Barriers to Classroom Performance*, Ph.D. thesis, Standford: Stanford University Press, p. 161.

[37]Johnson, Patrick (1983) *Native Children and the Child Welfare System*, Toronto: Canadian Council on Social Development and James Lorimer & Co., p. 23.

[38]Ibid.

[39]Fry, Alan (1970) *How A People Die*, New York: Tower Publications Inc., pp. 18-19.

[40]Government of Canada: Statement on Indian Policy, September 1969.

[41]Burke, J. (1976), *Paper Tomahawks: From Red Tape to Red Power*, Winnipeg: Queenston House, p. 23.

[42]It is only fair to note that this and other militant, public actions frequently caused some Indians, particularly many of the old people, embarrassment. While most agreed with the sentiment, 'they found this form of expression undignified. This particular sign has since been altered by graffiti artists to read "NIMPKISH INDIAN BAND," on the northward pointing arrow, and "NIMPKISH HOTEL," on the southward pointing arrow. It is interesting, however, to note that the sign remains standing, although a large cedar archway adorned by a local Indian artist's carved killer whale, commissioned and paid for by the Municipal Council, now competes with the shabby sign to greet people disembarking from the ferry.

[43]*Victoria Daily Colonist*, April 19, 1979.

[44]St. George's Hospital Society Constitution and By-Laws, as at 1979.

[45]Report presented to Municipal Council Meeting, Alert Bay, April 1974. Copy sent to Nimpkish Band Council.

[46]Nimpkish Band Council, public information package, distributed August 12, 1979.

[47]Ibid.

[48]Ibid.

CHAPTER 5

Did Renee Die
Because She Was An Indian?
The Inquest

*This is a court which is three hundred or four hundred years old,
but it is working even better in the twentieth century than it did in
the fourteenth or fifteenth centuries. If there is a pestilence in the land
and something is wrong, this is the forum where you have all the cover
of the judicial process for issuing subpoenaes and giving testimony
under oath....*

*So it is the kind of an open court where I think if we all go after
that point of view, perhaps at the end of the road we will have answered
the question Renee Smith would be maybe asking you, "How come
I am dead?"*

—Coroner Glen McDonald, LL.B.,
Supervising Coroner for B.C.

Alert Bay, B.C.
April-May, 1979

The inquest opened on April 18th in the lounge of Alert Bay's Royal Canadian Legion. It was abruptly adjourned the following day when, after a few

hours on the witness stand, and despite having been granted immunity from prosecution under the Canada Evidence Act, the St. George's nursing staff announced that they did not wish to proceed without legal counsel of their own.

"This looks much more than a routine inquest and we are requesting legal representation," the second nurse to take the stand told the Coroner.

During the five weeks of the adjournment "pro" and "anti" campaigns continued on both ends of town, and the media kept the controversy in the public eye. When hearings resumed on May 28, 1979, the proceedings were moved from the Legion to the Community Hall in order to accommodate the large number of lawyers, reporters, witnesses and spectators who had become involved.

The Supervising Coroner for B.C., Glen McDonald, two sheriffs and the court reporter sat at a long table facing the crowd. To the left of the coroner and the sheriffs sat the press, including reporters from the province's three daily papers, a national newspaper—the *Globe and Mail*, and the district weekly—the *North Island Gazette*. They were joined intermittently by camera crews and reporters from CBC and CTV National News.

Assembled in the first row facing them, on their left, were the lawyers everyone now referred to as "acting for the White End." These were attorneys representing Dr. Pickup; the St. George's Hospital Board, unregistered nurses and technicians; and the Registered Nurses. These men, members of prestigious law firms, seemed uncomfortably out of place in their three-piece, pin-striped suits amid the piles of floor hockey equipment and make-shift goal posts that had been hurriedly stacked in corners around the hall to make room for the proceedings. Seated with them was a young man, Sid Shook, who had recently been appointed prosecutor in nearby Campbell River. In this case, he was serving as the coroner's legal counsel.

Facing Coroner McDonald, on his right-hand side, were the lawyers acting for the "Indian side." Vancouver lawyer Michael Rhodes, hired by the Smith family, was dedicated and adept at his trade; but, in sharp contrast to the opposing lawyers, he showed little concern for keeping his shirt tucked in or his papers in order. Next to Rhodes sat the Nimpkish Band Council's lawyer, Rod Naknakin, a Native man from Campbell River who had just—that week— graduated from the University of British Columbia's Law School. Coroners holding inquests may, if they see fit, allow interested parties to have legal standing, including the right to cross-examine witnesses, and Coroner McDonald had granted such standing to the Nimpkish Band. Vera Robinson, the federal Indian Health Nurse, sat with Rhodes and Naknakin and acted as a consultant on details of medical and hospital procedures. Renee Taylor, a band member who was a law student at the time, and I, sat with the lawyers and acted as consultants on local details. Occasionally, members of the Nimpkish Band Council joined this table as well, as did the band's legal advisor of many years' standing, U.B.C. law professor Michael Jackson.

110

To the right of the coroner and the sheriffs, at their own table, sat the seven-person jury made up of two Native men, four non-Native men and one non-Native woman. Tom Wallace, a Band Councillor, and Danny Coon, a young artist, both came from the nearby Tsulquate Indian Reserve outside Port Hardy on Vancouver Island. The four non-Native men were John Goodchild, jury foreman and manager of a small retail outlet in Port McNeill; Greg Parnham, an auto mechanic also from Port McNeill; an accountant, Randy Brown, from Port Hardy, and a veterinarian, Andrew Rathewell from Coal Harbour. The only woman on the jury was Venitta Garner, a bank employee from Port McNeill.

Behind the lawyers' tables the spectators sat in rows of chairs and formed two distinct groups on either side of a central aisle. On the one side sat Indians and their supporters, and on the other side sat those who aligned themselves with the doctor and the hospital. While there were White people on the "Indian side" of the room, there were no Indians on the "White side" of the room. Occasionally, people from both communities entered, stood at the back of the hall, did not take a seat, and watched.

First to take the stand had been Dr. Colin Turnbull, former Campbell River radiologist, and veteran of fifty years' medical practice. Dr. Turnbull received, read, and returned reports on X-rays taken at St. George's. He testified that only chest X-rays were taken the day Renee was admitted to hospital with the diagnosis "acute abdomen." These films were taken on January 18th but Dr. Turnbull did not receive or interpret them until January 22nd, the day of her death. He explained that St. George's policy was to mail X-rays on Fridays only, and then they often take four days to reach Campbell River, 150 kilometres away. Yes, both towns do have a six-day-a-week mail delivery and pick-up service. Yes, St. George's is equipped with a new, modern X-ray unit and does have a full-time X-ray technician on staff. "As a rule," Dr. Turnbull testified, "the local doctor keeps X-rays while actively treating a patient and interprets them himself." In cases where the attending physician feels he requires a radiologist's opinion urgently, the X-rays are sent special delivery and the report returned by telex. Alternatively, telephone consultations are possible. No, he did not recall Dr. Pickup or anyone from St. George's contacting him by telephone to obtain the results of Renee's X-rays.

"Did...[this film]...show any congestion of the lungs?" Sid Shook asked.

"No," Dr. Turnbull replied.

"Did it show anything related to pneumonia?"

"No."

A second set of X-rays, this time of Renee's abdomen, were taken on Monday, January 22nd—the day of her death. They gave Dr. Turnbull "cause for concern" as some kind of bowel obstruction was indicated, but these films were not mailed out of Alert Bay until Friday, January 26th, and Dr. Turnbull did not receive and read them until January 30th, eight days after Renee died. Juror

Tom Wallace intervened and requested permission to question Dr. Turnbull.

"You work out of Campbell River?" Wallace asked.

"Yes," Dr. Turnbull answered.

"How busy are you?"

"I probably interpret up to seventy-five cases a day."

"Over an eight-hour day?"

"Yes."

"That is about approximately nine an hour?"

"Yes."

"So it is just like a factory?"

"Well, yes."

"Bang, bang, bang, hey? On this particular X-ray, did you have any real concern?"

"Yes, I was concerned."

"Were you concerned enough to make a note to phone the physician stating your concern?"

"I probably would but the films were taken on the 22nd and I saw them on the 30th, eight days later...and in the meantime the patient...I understood had been under the care of a competent physician and he hadn't required an immediate reply, so I don't know anything about the circumstances."

Coroner McDonald asked Dr. Turnbull about common practice in a case like Renee's. The doctor replied that Renee's symptoms appeared to be those commonly associated with appendicitis and, yes, he agreed that it was "relatively easy" to have a patient transferred from St. George's to a larger centre. He added, however, that he had specialized in radiology for the past forty years and had not performed any appendectomies since 1930.

Pressed by McDonald, Dr. Turnbull admitted that since "an appendix is a vestigial organ that is left over from our development and, in fact, has no exact function at the present time," very little had changed in the past forty years regarding diagnosis and treatment of appendicitis.

Reading from Tabor's Encyclopedic Medical Dictionary, McDonald read the list of symptoms of appendicitis: "'Abdominal pain, usually severe and generally throughout the abdomen...followed by nausea and vomiting, localization of pain in the right lower quadrant of abdomen with tenderness and rigidity over right rectus muscle'....Has this changed since 1930?" he asked Dr. Turnbull.

"No," the doctor replied.

Coroner McDonald continued: "'...fever usually rising within several hours from 37.2 to 38.2 degrees centigrade'...We have here the report of a temperature of 38.5...So we have the temperature..." Turning to recommended treatment, McDonald read on: "'...notify physician as soon as possible. Refrain from giving food, liquids, cathartic enemas and applying heat. Surgery as soon as the diagnosis is made is the safest procedure.' Do you agree?" he asked the witness.

"Yes," Dr. Turnbull replied.

McDonald then read Dr. Pickup's Discharge Summary, written February 1, 1979, ten days after Renee's death, into the court record:

"She was seen four times during the evening and early morning of January 18th and 19th with a view to emergency surgery. Then it became apparent that if she had an appendicitis, it had ruptured the day before and she already had general peritonitis. This and her chest condition made surgery a risky proposition and it was decided to treat her medically."

Next on the stand was Dr. Harmon, a pathologist with forty years' experience, who had performed the autopsy on Renee's body at Lion's Gate Hospital in North Vancouver. Margaret and Richard sat in the front row and listened silently as Dr. Harmon went through his pathologist's report in minute detail.

"The body is that of a well-nourished, well-developed American Indian female..." Dr. Harmon's report began. The deceased had been 5 feet 1 inch tall and had weighed 125 pounds. The body showed signs of dehydration—her eyes were sunken into her head. There was no evidence of any problem with her sexual organs. The lungs were not excessively heavy and showed no gross evidence of disease. Dr. Harmon proceeded to cite the weight of Renee's various organs and to list each and every part of her body which had been examined. Death had resulted, Dr. Harmon concluded, from generalized peritonitis from a ruptured appendix and the rupture of the appendix was the result of an acute gangrenous appendicitis.

Yes, he agreed, the incidence of death from a ruptured appendix in an eleven-year-old is very low nowadays. How low? Well, based on a computer search of the medical literature, Dr. Harmon estimated that "it could be as little as one in ten thousand...maybe even lower than that."

Pressed by Coroner McDonald for other results of his study of the literature regarding common practice, Dr. Harmon said "I believe most surgeons, the first thing they would look for in inflammation within the abdomen is the appendix....If the child's temperature is high; if the child is vomiting; pain within the side; problems with the bowel, then by and large you realize that you have something that looks pretty much like appendicitis condition."

What does the literature say about performing an operation when the diagnosis of appendicitis is only tentative, the coroner asked. Dr. Harmon replied, "...the general consensus is...the general consensus of surgical opinion is, if you can cut your ruptured appendixes to a lower percentage, it is better to subject some patients to unnecessary operations..."

Dr. Harmon believed that Renee's appendix had ruptured three or four days before her death, possibly before she came to the hospital, "but she was in a position to be operated on right up to the time of her death...something I believe should be treated at hospitals in major areas because it needs a surgical team approach." And as to operating after an appendix has already ruptured?

According to Dr. Harmon's research, 20-21 per cent of appendectomies are performed on ruptured appendixes. In determining whether to operate or to treat a patient medically, Dr. Harmon said "Close observation is a proper treatment in this particular instance."

Asked by Sid Shook about evidence of sexual assault, the doctor replied: "I was told by Staff Sergeant Barrie that there was some question that this girl had been sexually abused and I made a very thorough examination and found no evidence of any problem with her sexual organs. They were quite normal."

Dr. Pickup's lawyer rose to cross-examine Dr. Harmon. First, he concentrated on the weight of Renee's lungs.

"Doctor, you said that the normal or expected weight of a lung on autopsy was between 200 and 300 grams?" the lawyer queried.

"Yes."

"Is that for an adult?"

"Yes."

"How much would you expect the weight to be for a younger person?"

"25 per cent less."

"So then, the range for a normal eleven-year-old girl would run from 150 grams to approximately 200 to 250 grams?"

"Yes."

"On this young girl you weighed one lobe at 300 grams and the other at 400 grams?"

"Yes."

"On my calculation, Doctor, that is an increase of approximately 100 per cent over what you expect to be the normal or the anticipated weight of the lung size for a girl of that age?"

"No."

"Are you disagreeing with my percentages?"

"I am disagreeing with any conclusion that you may draw. I said her lungs were normal...it doesn't matter to me very much what the weight is. It could be twice what I found. In a person who dies of peritonitis and is very ill, I expect the lungs to be 600 to 700 grams in this age group. The lungs go up to 1500 to 2000 grams in disease...I don't know what you are getting at..."

"Don't worry what I am getting at, Doctor, just deal with the question. Each side weighed more than almost a 100 per cent or twice as much as a normal, well, eleven-year-old girl?"

"No." Dr. Harmon was clearly becoming exasperated with the lawyer's line of questioning.

"Well, Doctor, if you expect the weight of a well lung on one side to weigh between 150 grams and 200 grams and you weighed it and it is 300 and 400 grams, isn't that a variation of 100 per cent?" the lawyer persisted.

"Not over what I could expect to find...This is an eleven-year-old *ordinary* girl. This is a big girl for eleven years old..."

"Doctor, I am suggesting to you that the...condition of the lung tissue was consistent with a condition of aspiration pneumonia..."

"I just got through telling you she didn't have any pneumonia. There was nothing the matter with her lungs, so why bring this up? I was there. You weren't there...." Dr. Harmon snapped.

Dr. Pickup's lawyer then moved on to question Dr. Harmon's statement about a 1 in 10,000 incidence of death from appendicitis. Was it not true, he asked, that the risk of death increases if a patient delays seeking medical attention and waits until after the appendix has ruptured and peritonitis has set in? Yes, Dr. Harmon replied, the incidence of death in such cases increases to 1.8 in 10,000.

Finally, the lawyer raised the issue of multiple ailments confounding diagnosis.

"Doctor, what other conditions are there that present the practitioner with similar symptoms in a young girl of this age, as appendicitis? I suggest to you that an ectopic pregnancy...[is one]....Another one...[is]...a kidney abscess....Another...[is]...a perforated bowel....Another one is Meckel's diverticulitis....Another...[may be]...a perforated stomach....Another may be pelvic inflammatory disease?"

Dr. Harmon agreed that these conditions do present symptoms similar to those of appendicitis but when McDonald suggested adjourning to the following day when this line of questioning would be pursued further, Dr. Harmon objected angrily. "I want it to appear in the record that I don't see any reason for this fishing expedition that is going on this afternoon," he said.

Dr. Pickup's lawyer later admonished the pathologist. "There is an old adage, Doctor," the lawyer said sternly, "that one should be very careful before questioning a general out in the field in a war and I suggest to you that the medical practitioner who has the case, who is treating the case, is entitled to rely on his medical judgment as best he can on the facts he has....I am suggesting to you that patients can be difficult during the examination process and it makes it more difficult to carry out an examination. Do you agree with that?...And a patient who is unwilling to communicate or is poor in communication makes it more difficult for the practitioner to take a detailed history? And this would also hinder diagnosis. Do you agree with that?"

"Yes."

Under subsequent questioning from Smith family lawyer Michael Rhodes, Dr. Harmon agreed that, under normal circumstances, one does not place pregnancy high on the list of possible problems among eleven-year olds, particularly when, as was the case with Renee, the patient is menstruating during the time she is hospitalized. Furthermore, he added, a pregnancy test can be done in a hospital laboratory in approximately twenty minutes. Pelvic Inflammatory Disease is also more commonly found among older, sexually active women and can usually be diagnosed by pelvic and rectal examinations, neither of which Dr. Pickup conducted. Diagnosis of kidney abscesses is usually done by means of an abdominal X-ray, and such an X-ray was not taken until after Renee had been hospitalized for four days. A diagnosis of perforated bowel often requires exploratory surgery to be confirmed, and a stomach ulcer is most often found by ordering a barium study which takes twenty-four hours. Dr. Harmon agreed that in any case, four to five days was an unusually long period of observation to determine a diagnosis of such acute symptoms.

Finally, Dr. Harmon was asked again, by Rhodes, about evidence of sexual assault. He replied, again, that he had found no evidence whatsoever to substantiate that allegation. He read aloud from Renee's medical history. "'As a child she fell off a tree branch and a foreign body hit her thigh near the vagina while she was going to school and this occurred on September 20, 1973 at 12:15 at the Alert Bay School grounds.' But there was no recent injury and no suggestion of sexual assault."

Leonard Smith, Renee's uncle who had been looking after her and her younger brother while their parents were on vacation, took the stand. A young man in his early thirties, Leonard described the events which led up to his bringing Renee to the hospital the first time. The children had both had colds when their parents left on Thursday, January 11th. Leonard had taken them to see Dr. Pickup on Saturday, January 13th, at which time cough medicine and pills were prescribed. Renee and Richard Jr. had stayed home on Monday, the 15th, but both had returned to school on Tuesday, the 16th. On Wednesday, January 17th, Renee complained of pains in her stomach and Leonard kept her home from school again. By the end of the day, the pains had worsened, he had become worried, and had decided to take her to the hospital.

"I phoned before I brought her down and explained the problem and they told me to bring her down," Leonard said.

At the hospital, he had seen a nurse whose name he could not remember. He identified her only as "one of the Filipino nurses." He didn't talk to her about Renee's problem. "I just told them she was in bad pain. They could see in her expression she could hardly walk. I had to hold her up."

Dr. Pickup's lawyer appeared to find it incredible that Leonard had not discussed Renee's symptoms in detail with the nurse. "You brought your eleven-year-old niece in to the hospital to have her looked at and you said to the nurse...words to the effect, 'Here is my niece, she is having some trouble with her stomach'...that's all?"

"Yep," Leonard replied.

The nurse on duty had taken Renee into a private examining room and had told Leonard to wait outside, to pay the two-dollar emergency fee, and to sign the out-patient forms which the admitting clerk had completed. Dr. Pickup's lawyer questioned Leonard about the nurse's notation on this form, which read "general abdominal pain since yesterday." Leonard said he had told the nurse he spoke to on the phone that Renee had been sick for a few days but that the pains in her stomach had only been bad since that morning.

"I suggest to you that you are not really sure when the pains started, are you?" Dr. Pickup's lawyer barked.

"It was in the morning," Leonard replied.

"You don't remember which day it was," the lawyer continued.

"I certainly do. It was Wednesday, the 17th," Leonard insisted. Renee had gone to school the day before, Tuesday the 16th.

Renee had emerged from the examining room about fifteen minutes later with some pills. Leonard had taken her home and, as she was even worse the following morning, Thursday, the 18th, he had phoned Mrs. Pickup, told her what was wrong and had been given an appointment for 4:30 p.m., at which time Renee had been admitted to hospital by Dr. Pickup with a diagnosis of "acute abdomen." The out-patient form said that Leonard had been "advised to see doctor in the A.M.," but Leonard denied having been told to do this and claimed he had made the appointment on his own initiative. Again, Dr. Pickup's lawyer took issue with Leonard's account:

"I am suggesting to you, Mr. Smith, that you didn't state to the person on the other end of the telephone that...[the appointment]...was for stomach pains."

"I did state it," Leonard responded, "because I had to. There was no other choice. When they ask you, you have to tell them what the appointment is for."

A great deal of confusion then arose about the forms Leonard had signed when Renee was admitted to the hospital. Both the out-patient form and the admitting form listed two clauses over a single signature, one of which stated that the signatory to the form was giving permission for medical treatment and the other stipulating that consent was also given for necessary surgery. Leonard had signed such a form on the 17th, and again on the 18th when Renee was finally admitted. A line appeared to have been drawn through the "consent to surgery" portion of the admitting form. Leonard said he had signed forms on both evenings, but he hadn't read either of them. He had simply told them he couldn't consent to surgery and had then signed where the nurses had told him to.

Coroner McDonald tried to sort this out. "Did you sign that document there?" he demanded, showing Leonard the double consent form.

"I did," Leonard said.

"And do you know what that document says? You are giving consent to a surgical operation?" McDonald continued.

"Well, I didn't read this...." Leonard explained.

"But you had given consent on the 17th and then there was some discussion the next day, on the 18th, when you couldn't give consent and they crossed it out?...So, actually, they took your signature on here without you understanding that it was a consent for treatment and/or operation?" McDonald asked.

"I guess they could have," Leonard responded.

"Anyway...this is your signature?" growled McDonald.

"Yes. But I didn't give no consent. That is for sure I didn't." Leonard was calm, but adamant.

"Well, why did you sign your name then?" McDonald snapped.

"I don't know how they work it...But...I told them...I just signed where they said to sign, but I never signed for an operation."

Leonard would not be budged.

"Are you saying that you did not sign and that is not your signature?" McDonald demanded.

"I am not saying that or anything. I am just saying that I didn't give no consent at all...I didn't sign no papers for consent for Renee to be operated on, until I got word from the parents. That's what I told all of them....Pickup and the nurses," Leonard insisted.

Leonard had given the R.C.M.P. a statement when they had interrogated him for four hours after the administrator, the staff sergeant, the doctor and the mortician believed they had found evidence of Renee having been sexually assaulted. Two weeks later, when the petitions requesting an inquest into Renee's death and an inquiry into the hospital had begun circulating, the Smith family had contacted their lawyer, who had suggested that they each try to write out everything they remembered about the events surrounding the death, before the details faded from memory. Leonard explained that he had gone to the R.C.M.P. and asked for a copy of his statement but that they had refused to give it to him, even though the results of the autopsy were in and any question of sexual abuse had been dismissed. (Coroner McDonald advised him that he did have a right to see his statement and that he could not understand why the R.C.M.P. had kept it from him.) Leonard then wrote out a new statement and asked his ex-wife to type it.

Dr. Pickup's lawyer seized upon minor discrepancies between the two statements. The language in the second statement, he insinuated, was not Leonard's.

"I suggest to you that some of the things contained in it are not your recollection but they are a reconstruction of events," the lawyer began.

"Some of the words were rephrased," Leonard agreed.

"'...Transportation to and from the movie theatre was by taxi.' That is a sentence that was rephrased," the lawyer continued, reading from Leonard's second statement. "You didn't say '...Transportation to and from...'"

"Yes," Leonard answered. "I just say '...we took a cab to the show...'"

"So," Dr. Pickup's lawyer said triumphantly, "this document that you described as your statement yesterday, prepared by yourself, is not one that you made up yourself, is it?"

"I made up the statement but she just rephrased it. After she typed it, I just went over it. She put the different wordings into it. That's all," Leonard said.

"She rewrote it. That's what you say? She changed the wording didn't she?" Dr. Pickup's lawyer persisted.

"It was my statement in the first place, but it was just reworded. She's better at that...you know...English...and the right words...than me....so she just put some different words in," Leonard explained matter-of-factly.

"Then why did you say it was your statement that you made, Mr. Smith.... Yesterday you said that you wrote this statement, that you wrote it out and it was your statement," the lawyer went on.

"Yes," Leonard replied.

"And that's not true?" the lawyer pushed.

Coroner McDonald intervened and called a short recess to allow Leonard time to review both of his statements. The one recorded by the R.C.M.P. on January 25th said that after Renee was admitted to hospital on the 18th, Leonard had called his brother, Richard, in Reno and had told him that Dr. Pickup had said that Renee's appendix "might have to come out soon." In the statement he wrote on February 9th, Leonard said that Dr. Pickup had told him that Renee "would have to be operated on immediately."

"The statements are more or less the same... It's still what I said... I advised them—Richard and Margaret—that Renee might have to be operated on. But I didn't know...[if]...she was going to be operated on or not. But Pickup said she has to be operated on right away," Leonard stated when he resumed the stand.

Leonard was questioned extensively on his activities during the period of time Renee had been in his care. Where had he gone during those eight days? Who else had been in the home? Had he been drinking? Had any other young men been at the house?

Leonard hadn't done much of anything. Everyone was pretty broke after Christmas. The weather in January is wet and cold. He'd had two sick kids on his hands. He'd watched a lot of T.V. He had not gone out—except to do household errands. He had not had visitors. He had not been drinking.

Didn't he think his niece was very mature—physically—for her age?

She was pretty big, he guessed.

But didn't he find her *sexually* mature?

Well, he was her uncle, how would he know about things like *that*?

Some people on the "White" side of the room smirked and exchanged meaningful glances. Indians tensed, clenched their jaws and stared straight ahead. The lawyers hammered away at Leonard about how he felt when the police picked him up in the middle of the night and interrogated him.

"I was upset," Leonard replied.

Was he upset because of the allegations being made about sexual assault? Leonard responded quietly that it was his niece's death that had upset him.

"I loved my niece," he said, meeting the lawyer's gaze directly.

The questioning lawyer glanced pointedly at the jury and returned to his seat. Leonard was dismissed from the witness stand and went back to sit next to Richard and Margaret who blinked back tears and nodded solemnly to him.

Other people reached over and affectionately squeezed his arm or patted his shoulder. No one said a word, but the dignified manner with which Leonard had endured this questioning was acknowledged by the "Indian side" of the hall.

People in Alert Bay watch a lot of T.V., including many popular "cops and lawyers shows." It seemed obvious that the lawyers for the White End were trying to "plant the seeds of doubt" in the minds of the jury members and the media. Everyone was familiar with the images they were exploiting to obtain these objectives.

First of all, they appeared to be trying to paint a picture of Leonard as being incompetent and unreliable so as to make it seem that by the time Renee had been brought to the doctor, it was too late. Secondly, they attempted to bring out evidence to support the theory that diagnosis had been confounded by her general ill health, or by other specific ailments. Thirdly, they emphasized the fact that her parents had been away at the time she became ill and suggested that her home life was disorganized. Fourthly, they continually, in various ways, raised sexual innuendos. Renee may have been eleven but she was mature, *sexually* mature. No innocent child here. Keep raising the already thoroughly discredited allegation of sexual abuse. Hint at incest. Keep this alive. Reinforce with the idea that pregnancy was a possible diagnosis.

The lawyers for the "Indian side" had said that "the other side" would not be concerned with the inquest itself but would view it as preliminary to potential civil negligence suits and would therefore concentrate on ensuring that appropriate themes were reflected in the transcript. They appeared to be pursuing a classic strategy for a legal defence against medical negligence: patient responsibility.

Until the 1960s medical authority was essentially unchallenged by most people, even those who had not experienced its imposition in as dramatic and thorough a manner as Native peoples had. Questioning doctors was simply not done, and was certainly not encouraged by doctors themselves who jealously guarded their exclusive knowledge and skills. With the general upsurge in "consumer awareness" in many areas, doctors' power and authority began to be questioned publicly, and, most significantly, in the courts, as malpractice suits became the bane of the medical profession.

According to Lorne Rozovsky, author of *Canadian Hospital Law* (2nd edition):

> The relationship between the patient and the health facility and its staff has two bases. One is a contract either express or implied. The other is that the facility and the staff have held themselves out as being capable of providing particular services at a reasonable level....The relationship therefore consists of a duty to the patient and the right of the patient to that duty....

The only occasion in which the patient's duty arises is as part of a lawsuit brought by the patient usually on the grounds of negligence. The issue of the patient's duty is brought up by the defendant (doctor) as a defence....

In the case of a total defence, the defendant (doctor) is saying that the injury to the patient was not caused by the defendant (doctor). It was caused solely by the patient....

The partial defence of patient duty is raised in answer to a clearly established allegation of negligence. The defence is that the injury was not totally caused by the negligence of the defendant. It was partially caused by the patient.[1]

Lawyers are hired to win specific cases. In order to achieve this, they generally pursue a two-pronged strategy. On the one hand they muster evidence to argue points of law: did their client's actions contravene specific laws or not? On the other hand, they strive to convince judges and juries that their client is not the *type of person* who breaks the law, and/or that the person making the complaint against their client is not the *type of person* whose statements should be given any credibility.

In Renee Smith's particular case, Dr. Pickup's lawyers, and the lawyers for the hospital and its staff, apparently relied on the specific characteristics usually attributed to Native patients (See BCMA Federal/Provincial Indian Health Committee Report, 1970, Chapter 4, pp. 98-99): Renee had presented herself too late. Her appendix had already ruptured. She masked her symptoms because of her high tolerance for pain, her stoicism. She had been unco-operative and uncommunicative. Her general ill health had complicated the diagnosis. (Although the only diagnosis ever made by Dr. Pickup was "acute abdomen," which, in layman's terms, is equivalent to "bad stomach ache.") Her parents were away. Her relatives wouldn't obey rules. There was the confounding issue of suspected, possibly incestuous, sexual abuse.

Now, how were Renee's family and other members of the Native community to know that these were abstract legal strategies? To them, it seemed that the lawyers were simply repeating the kinds of things they had seen written on the walls of public toilets. It was grossly insulting. Of course, the lawyers were only doing their jobs, earning their very concrete fees. The real problem was that they were playing to a receptive audience. Judges and juries composed of ordinary Canadian citizens would find all this palatable.

The Filipino-Canadian Graduate Nurse who had seen Renee the first time Leonard had brought her to the hospital on the evening of January 17th testified next. Referring to notes she had written a week to ten days afterwards, she recounted what had taken place, claiming that Renee had told her then that "she had the stomach pain on and off, but *yesterday* ...[the *16th*]...was the worst." The nurse insisted that she had explained to Leonard that Dr. Pickup wanted Renee to stay in the hospital that night and that she had told him to call the doctor's office for an appointment the next morning. She emphasized that Renee wouldn't co-operate when she tried to examine her and that she swore at her and said "I don't have to stay in this damned hospital." "She say 'Just give me pain killer. I am in pain,'" the nurse testified, adding that Renee told her she was menstruating and that this led her to assume the girl was suffering from menstrual cramps.

Coroner McDonald, a large and overbearing man with a bushy mane of white hair and a loud gruff voice interjected impatiently. "Who runs this hospital? Is it an eleven-year-old girl who says she won't be a patient after a doctor has ordered her to be admitted? Or is it a silent uncle? Or who does? She just walks in, picks up pills under prescription and takes them home, like jelly beans, I suppose? And just eats them? Or is the uncle supposed to be in charge of that procedure, do you know? You see, at some stage of the game this girl is a child, or she is an adult. She is certainly not an adult...In the Philippines, would an eleven-year-old girl be able to walk into a hospital and walk out on her own?"

"Normally the girl goes with parents," the nurse answered.

"Would an uncle not be acceptable?"

"He would be acceptable if he would sign the consent."

"But the consent was signed. We've just been over that."

"Yes."

"Why was that not acted upon? You have Renee. You have the uncle's signature. You have the doctor's name. You have a bed ready for her. Here we have a doctor saying one thing and an eleven-year-old child saying I won't go. How come this girl says what happens to her when the hospital has a consent form signed by a legal guardian?" McDonald bellowed.

"I don't know," the nurse whispered .

"I don't know either," McDonald snarled.

Results of blood and urine tests taken when Renee was admitted were not completed by the hospital laboratory until four days later, on the day of her death. The nurse didn't know why. It was crucial, she agreed, that an input/output chart with daily fluid balance totals be kept on a patient with symptoms like those displayed by Renee. No such record had been kept for January 18, 19, 20 or 22. It had been done on the 21st. The nurse didn't know why this had happened.

Under questioning by the Smith family's lawyer, the nurse admitted that Renee had been given medication for four days without the benefit of a doctor's diagnosis and that this was not considered normal procedure in most hospitals. She had been "concerned but not upset" about the lack of a diagnosis, although she confessed this was the first time in her five-year nursing career that she had seen a patient being treated for so long without a specific diagnosis. At

St. George's, she said, orders are frequently written by the Head Nurse and then signed by the doctor. She denied that the nurses had discussed Renee's case among themselves.

The nurse testified that she had been working at St. George's since July 1978 and had never witnessed Dr. Pickup treating patients while under the influence of alcohol.

Next to take the stand was the Registered Nurse who had admitted Renee to St. George's on January 18th. Defensive and defiant, she requested protection under the Canada Evidence Act before testifying. "I am not a doctor. I am sorry. I am just a nurse and at that a very plain one....I can only do what the doctor writes down as to medicine....I am only the nurse. We are only trained to fulfill procedures," she told the inquest.

The Admitting Nurse listed the procedures she had followed in admitting Renee to the hospital on January 18th. She was most reluctant, however, to reveal what she had recorded in her "confidential nurse's notes" about questions she had asked Renee that night, and argued for some time with McDonald about this issue. Finally, the Coroner put his foot down. "This child died in a public place with persons who were paid by the public and I think that the public are entitled to hear it."

The notes the nurse wished not to place in the record read as follows: "...patient states she felt chills three days ago. She had epigastric pain starting yesterday—or—since yesterday...[the *17th*]...which are now very strong. Breathing is easy."

Asked how she determined correct dosages of medication to be administered to Renee since she did not weigh her, the Admitting Nurse said she had guessed at her weight and taken it from there. Challenged on such guesswork by Rod Naknakin, the Nimpkish Band's lawyer, she replied haughtily that he would be surprised if she told him his weight. "Go ahead," he said. The nurse looked Mr. Naknakin over. "One hundred and fifty pounds," she declared triumphantly. "You're out by about twenty-five pounds," the lawyer replied.

Three drugs were given to Renee while she was hospitalized: an adult dosage of the narcotic Sparidol; Dramamine to combat nausea, and penicillin. "I assumed from my observations Renee was a probably acute appendicitis case and it was my impression when I saw her two days after she was admitted she had moved from an acute to a chronic appendix case," the Admitting Nurse testified.

Had she been concerned about the fact that there was no diagnosis? Yes, but she couldn't recall whether or not she had mentioned this concern to any other nurses or to the doctor.

She testified for three hours, admitting that she had expressed concern to Dr. Pickup about Renee's constant vomiting and suggested to him that he change from oral antibiotics to intravenous.

This nurse was particularly agitated about the number of visitors Renee had received. "A lot of visitors she had. Not one. Not two. Not three. A lot! It seems to be forever people coming in. Some people came in dragging a T.V......I remember going once in there and asking one visitor at a time only and I put a note on the door saying to refer to the Nurse's Station first before entering the room..." she complained.

She also said Renee had been unco-operative and apprehensive when Dr. Pickup had come in to examine her, but she found nothing objectionable about her behaviour in this regard. "An eleven-year-old girl, just on the break of puberty," the nurse said, "those are very healthy signs to me....I asked her who is the most significant person in her life and she tells me it was her mother.... Renee was a very shy girl and I tried to assure her....In my opinion, I think this is very good for a young girl in this day and age, your Honour."

However, when asked about the absence of a fluid balance total for four out of the five days Renee had been hospitalized, and the unusually few number of visits Dr. Pickup appeared to have paid to this patient, the nurse flew off the handle. "I can't answer for the other shift....I can only answer for what I observed...I love you people that like bureaucracy. It is really fantastic! It is absolutely incredible! I am a nurse and although the records have been—my patient's condition is more concern to me than all the bureaucracies in between....If I have to worry about all these things while trying to nurse the patient properly, you would have the nurse behind the desk and none on the bedside....I can assure you by the whole truth and nothing but the truth that he has seen her more often than there is stated."

Leo O'Connell, mortician, took the stand next and described in lurid detail his encounter with Dr. Pickup, Mrs. Pickup, the R.C.M.P. Staff Sergeant, and the hospital administrator the night he had begun to prepare Renee's body for burial and had become uneasy about the possibility of rape and about the absence of a signed death certificate specifying cause of death. His testimony raised the Coroner's ire once again. "What were you thinking of when you began embalming procedures without a death certificate? I don't know how a deceased person can be approached without first obtaining an official order," McDonald thundered.

O'Connell's evidence also marked a turning point in the media's treatment of the inquest. Up to this point, articles had been appearing on first and second pages of the province's daily papers under headlines such as "Nurses Balk at Alert Bay Inquest." Now, however, a banner headline proclaimed "DEATH PROBE TOLD DOCTOR DRUNK: WITNESS."

R.C.M.P. Staff Sergeant Barrie was called to the stand and Mr. Naknakin cross-examined him.

Was it true that Dr. Pickup was intoxicated at the morgue the night he attended there with the doctor, the administrator, and the mortician?

The sergeant couldn't say as he had not run sobriety tests on the doctor.

If the doctor had been in command of an automobile would he have allowed him to continue driving?

No, he would not have.

Did it concern him that the only doctor on the island, who was on call at the hospital, was too drunk to drive a car?

No, it did not.

Is protecting the public part of his responsibilities?

Yes, it is.

Did he think he had been derelict in his duty that night?

No, he did not.

Next, Dr. Pickup took the stand. When he first saw Renee, he said, he thought she had pneumonia. "I told the uncle there was a possibility an operation would be necessary as a lever to get him to agree the girl remain in hospital." So he knew that if her uncle told her to stay in the hospital she would have done so. Why had he not done this the first night she came to the hospital? He didn't know.

He had considered operating on her every day but her chest condition made that proposition risky. The medication given Renee "seemed what was required at the time."

Later on, Dr. Pickup said he had assumed that Renee had the flu. "I was never able to localize the condition so I could diagnose the problem," he said. "But I suspected general peritonitis or the flu. I considered operating on her every day. At no time did I get a definite reading. Her general condition was such that an operation was a risk." [*Complications in treatment occur because many Indians have multiple ailments and also because their general health is poor.*[2]]

"In retrospect, I feel Renee's appendix ruptured the day before she entered hospital," Dr. Pickup testified. [*Indian patients fail to recognize early symptoms of illness...Indian patients present in the acute and often fatal stages of an illness.*[3]]

He, too, complained that Renee had pushed his hand away when he had begun examining her and noted that she "masked her pain." [*They have a higher tolerance for pain and discomfort.*[4]]

Dr. Pickup said he refused Renee's parents', aunts' and grandfather's requests that she be flown to a larger hospital because weather conditions in January made travel dangerous. [*And a fatalistic acceptance of things as they are...*[5]]

Rhodes obtained weather reports for January 18-22 from the Department of Transport weather station in Alert Bay. Flying was possible each day and night, with the exception of a period of approximately one hour around 4:00 a.m., January 20th.

"Looking at the situation in hindsight," Dr. Pickup said, "I would have operated on the first night she was in hospital or would have had her transferred to another hospital next day."

125

He had thought it might be appendicitis at one point but Renee had refused to let him do the rectal examination necessary to diagnose appendicitis. Had he asked any of the many female relatives who were in constant attendance to persuade Renee to allow this examination? No, he hadn't.

Yes, there had been a staff party going on at his house on the evening of January 17th when Leonard had first brought Renee to the hospital, but he'd only had two drinks.

Yes, he had attended another party the following night, January 18th, when Renee was admitted, but he had only taken one drink on that occasion.

Yes, he admitted, he had had several drinks on the afternoon of Renee's death, the 22nd, "...but I don't recall if I had drinks after supper—but I doubt it. I thought she was getting better. That's why I had a drink," the doctor testified.

Yes, he had had "a few" on the night of the 24th when he, the mortician, the administrator, and the R.C.M.P. officers had gone to the morgue, but he denied that his mind was clouded by alcohol. Asked if he could say how much alcohol he consumed in an average day or an average week, Dr. Pickup said he couldn't give figures but "I never considered myself to be an alcoholic."

Why had he not entered a cause of death on the death certificate? "I wasn't sure why she died. I thought it was pulmonary," he said.

He reiterated his position that he had not contacted the local coroner and was opposed to an autopsy because the girl's family did not want one. "Autopsies are not popular with families in general and it's my impression the native people are very opposed to them." Someone, he couldn't remember exactly who, had told him that Renee's family specifically did not want an autopsy in this case.

Dr. Pickup maintained that Renee's vaginal scarring was consistent with injuries which resulted from rape. His examination of the body in the morgue revealed that Renee's vagina had been injured sometime earlier and repaired by a doctor, he said. The Smith's lawyer, Michael Rhodes, attempted to clarify how a *previously* treated, and healed, injury could be mistaken for evidence of a very *recent* rape. Dr. Pickup stood his ground. "The injury could have been mistaken for sexual assault," he insisted.

The doctor testified that his reluctance to report this to the police came from his concern for the feelings of the family, who, he said, "had been through enough grief already."

Explaining differences involved in treating Indian patients, Dr. Pickup said "There's the language, culture and background that are important." However, he said that he had not treated Renee any differently because she was an Indian.

Regarding the absence of any patient history and the serious omissions and discrepancies in other medical records that had been brought to light by the nurses' testimonies, Dr. Pickup admitted he was responsible but said that he had had no holiday in eighteen months and was on seven-day-a-week, twenty-four-hour call at the hospital since he had been the only doctor on the island for nearly a year now and was too overburdened to worry about paperwork. Anyway, he said, "on the whole our records are pretty reliable."

The Head Nurse testified that it was not totally unusual for it to take four days to obtain results from the hospital laboratory. She didn't know why exactly, but the lab was closed on Saturdays and sometimes on Wednesday. Shown a copy of Renee's hospital file and asked why input/output and fluid balance sheets were not kept up, she said she didn't know. The nurses were responsible for chart work and she assumed she was responsible for making sure the nurses did their jobs. "I don't really know what happened on these occasions," she said. She had noticed that Renee never received a diagnosis but had assumed that she had the flu. The Head Nurse could not recall whether or not any of the nurses had asked her why Renee's condition had not been diagnosed. At no time did Renee's illness strike her as "exceedingly serious."

Another nurse testified that all the nurses had been talking about Renee's condition. "All the indications were that something was very wrong with her," she said. It was the day shift who had neglected to maintain input/output charts. She was on night shift. [*Apathy, I think is the best way to describe what happens to medical personnel charged with the health maintenance of Indians. It is a creeping complacency catching the most committed professional. It takes hold. It is dangerous.*[6]]

One after another, the witnesses for the "White side" took the stand and, either glaring defiantly at the "Indian side" of the room or mumbling with downcast eyes, responded to the questions put before them. On the Indian side, people, including Renee's parents, sat and listened, eyes rivetted on the witnesses, silent tears occasionally streaking their faces as Renee's illness and death were relived in clinical detail. On the "White side" of the hall Dr. Pickup's supporters sat, lips pursed and eyes staring straight ahead. Day after day, old familiar themes shaped the testimonies of witnesses for the "White side."

All the nurses denied that the doctor had ever been at the hospital while under the influence of alcohol. At some point in their testimonies, most of the nurses, often addressing meaningful glances to the coroner, raised the following issues: The child's parents were out of town, you know— in Reno! They had had a good deal of trouble controlling the number of visitors in Renee's room—no one would listen. [*Before being taught by the missionaries, Indians lacked our idea of a moral sensibility and that fine feeling which we commonly call sentiment. Their ideas seemed very gross as compared to the Christian ideals....*[7]]

The girl had been rude to the doctor and the nurses and had been uncooperative. Someone had heard her say, in her sleep, "Don't touch me any more." They suspected sexual abuse. [*Children were rarely rebuked....girls were sold to the highest bidder....they have been mortgaged for potlatch debts before they were five years old....*[8]]

127

Rhodes and Naknakin pursued these issues. Were the nurses aware of the Louisa James case?

They'd heard things.

Were they aware of the fact that Louisa was Renee's aunt?

Well, they're all related it seems.

Did they think Renee's apparent rudeness could have resulted from fear?

They hadn't thought of that.

Was Reno not a popular holiday spot?

Yes.

Did a lot of people not go to Reno?

Yes.

Is it not common for parents to go away on short vacations alone and to arrange to place their children in the care of relatives while they are away?

Yes.

Did this constitute child neglect?

Well...no...It depends.

Were the relatives who visited Renee rude?

No, not really, they just didn't listen.

Could this have been caused by their concern about her condition?

Yes, I suppose so.

Were the visiting relatives ever asked to persuade Renee to be more co-operative?

No.

Were the nurses' suspicions regarding sexual assault based only on Renee's alleged mutterings in her sleep?

Yes.

They had not heard any gossip about a suspicion of sexual assault?

No....Well...maybe.

Did they socialize with RCMP officers?

Yes. Sometimes.

Had they heard it there?

No, definitely not.

The lawyers for Dr. Pickup and the hospital called a general practitioner, Dr. Leslie Patterson, as an expert witness to testify as to what constitutes "common practice."

Dr. Patterson began his testimony by saying that he, like Dr. Pickup, was "overburdened with a fear that Renee Smith had reached the point of no return before she was admitted to St. George's on January 18th....I would say she was a goner on the 18th."

Mr. Rhodes pointed out that fifty-one appendectomies had been performed at St. George's Hospital since 1968, sixteen of these had been operations performed on ruptured appendixes and Renee's had been the only death.

Dr. Patterson expressed his admiration for the courage shown by this "little girl who so bravely masked her pain."

He criticized Dr. Pickup for prescribing pain killers, for not visiting Renee immediately after she was admitted to the hospital, and for not performing a rectal examination. "I would have gone over and tried to mollify this lovely little girl. I would have done a rectal examination even if it meant having to give her an anaesthetic to do it. It's fundamental to the diagnosis," Dr. Patterson testified. But, he maintained, "her chest condition would have killed her under general anaesthetic."

Dr. Patterson then went on to argue that Renee's refusal to carry out a doctor's orders to be admitted to hospital "abrogated any contract between doctor and patient." Rhodes corrected the doctor's interpretation of the law regarding children and contracts, pointing out that doctors do not require a contractual arrangement before treating an eleven-year-old and, furthermore, that if a contract had been breached, Dr. Pickup, by prescribing pain killers, had re-established the contract. Dr. Patterson deferred to lawyer Rhodes on this point.

The doctor then proceeded to argue that although Renee, that "lovely little girl" he had been referring to, was eleven years old *chronologically*, "she was an adult in every sense." He cited her height, weight, "metabolism" and the fact that she had begun menstruating. He agreed with Rhodes that age sixteen is usually the youngest age at which anyone is ever considered to be an adult in any sense, and that eleven seemed a ways from sixteen, but Dr. Patterson insisted nonetheless that Renee was in a "grey area."

Dr. Leslie Patterson admitted that he had an "inherent desire" to protect another doctor.

The press, while having sensed a whopper of a story from the very beginning, had been somewhat sceptical about all the charges the Indians were making. However, after the first week of testimony by the hospital staff and Dr. Pickup, scepticism had turned to incredulity and the contrast between the warm, hospitable, grieving family, and the hostile, tight-lipped Pickup supporters—who had made the error of refusing to speak to the press—had polarized the reporters' sympathies. They filed their stories, and their editors gave them front-page space and sensational headlines. Panoramic shots of the graveyard's tall totems casting eerie shadows over the old wooden hospital on the water's edge, and Dr. and Mrs. Pickup hurrying along the road to their bungalow after each day's proceedings, became a regular clip on the T.V. news of both national networks.

The editor of the *North Island Gazette*, Peter Paterson, was moved to write a second editorial in his weekly column, "Left Field," responding, a few weeks after the fact, to the criticisms he had received for his "Curs snapping at the heels of an old warrior" piece. The inquest, it seemed, had encouraged Mr. Paterson to rethink his choice of words:

...my peculiarly gyrating mind has swung closer to home and it is time to attempt to set straight something I wrote several weeks ago....

I wrote about 'those few who have instigated such a disproportionately furious attack upon Dr. Pickup...' Not for an instant did it occur to me that the 'handful' and the 'few' would be misread to mean the whole of the hundreds of members of the Nimpkish Indian Band.

....I do not consider an inquest to be an attack, it is a perfectly proper legal institution, so nowhere in my criticism of the degree of the attack upon Pickup did any of the inquest witnesses or even the family of Renee Smith enter the picture.... To the members of the Nimpkish Indian Band who have written to me or spoken to me on the matter, I repeat, I am sorry you took my words so broadly, they were not meant for you.

Next, members of Renee's family testified. Relatives brought urns full of coffee and plugged them in at the back of the hall. Women arrived with platters of home-baked cakes and tarts. This was an important public event. The truth would be told, and witnessed, and the Kwakwaka'wakw always feed their guests well.

Arthur Dick, Sr., Renee's grandfather, was asked about the days leading up to her death. Prior to this incident Mr. Dick and Dr. Pickup had been friends, of sorts. Because they were both successful men in their chosen fields and leaders of their respective communities, it was not unheard of for them to join one another at the Legion on a Friday night to share a drink or two while discussing local events. Even a man who shared the doctor's table at the Legion, however, could not have his granddaughter transferred out of St. George's.

"I've seen a lot in my day," Arthur Dick, Sr. explained. "My grand-daughter, that day before her death, she—her eyes were sunken right into her head. She was in great pain and she was very sick child. I know that. That's why I try to talk to Jack about moving her to a big place. He just told me she had bad stomach flu."

What was the feeling of his family regarding an autopsy? Are Indians opposed to autopsies as a rule? The old man paused to consider the question, and then responded. "In my family when someone dies, we wait for the RCMP to come tell us if there's going to be autopsy or not."

Renee's father, Richard, recounted in detail the last evening of his daughter's life. When asked about Renee's now nationally famous vaginal scars, Richard explained that when Renee was about six years old she had been playing in the woods behind the school and had fallen, injuring herself. A teacher had taken Renee to St. George's where the injury had been treated with stitches.

Renee's aunts testified about the time they had spent in the hospital with her. No, she had not been alone at any time, except when they had been asked by the nurses to wait outside her room while they administered various treatments. No, they had never heard her cry out a man's name. Yes, they had been there when she died. "The sight of Dr. Pickup massaging my niece's heart in an attempt to revive her with a cigar sticking out of the corner of his mouth really upset me," Eva Cook testified.

Next, Michael Rhodes called expert witnesses. Vera Robinson, the federal Indian Health Nurse, had worked at a clinic for Native people in North Battle-ford, Saskatchewan, and she had contacted the physicians there, who agreed to come to Alert Bay on short-term locum arrangements to run the Band Clinic which Medical Services had equipped and furnished, but had been unable to staff with a doctor. Dr. Alan Gonar, a General Practitioner, and Dr. June Mills, an internist, had arrived in town from Saskatchewan in early May.

First to take the stand was Dr. Mills, who began her testimony by explain-ing that she had had extensive experience working for Medical Services in Indian communities all over Canada and that she had reviewed all the hospital records pertaining to Renee's treatment and subsequent death. On this basis, she said, she could state unequivocally that Renee's death had not been inevitable.

She criticized the treatment Renee had received and said that on a scale of one to ten, with "one" as the lowest, Renee's care deserved a "two" and "reached the level of malpractice." Specifically, Mills listed as unacceptable procedures both the nurses' and the doctor's examinations, the absence of a rectal examination, inadequate X-rays, incorrect nurses' charting, incorrect drugs, and empty oxygen tanks. She argued that patients should never be sent home with acute abdominal pains and that "the basic problem in this case was the absence of a rectal examination. There's no substitute. It is essential." Furthermore, the whole charting procedure was incorrect and the continued administration of high doses of narcotic pain-killers served to mask Renee's symptoms, which were clearly those of appendicitis.

As to the patient being unco-operative, Dr. Mills noted that in a situation where there is a doctor with thirty years of practice behind him, several ex-perienced nurses and countless relatives in attendance, this "should not have been a problem." Had she been in charge, she said, she would have insured that Renee was admitted to the hospital on January 17th, when she was first presented there. Immediately following admission, Dr. Mills said, she would have obtained legal consent to operate whether this was done by persuading Renee's uncle, Leonard, to authorize it, or by obtaining the signature of one other doctor, or the hospital administrator. She then would have conducted a thorough examination, including a rectal, and taken lab tests and X-rays. Had these normal procedures been followed, there should have been little if any problem in diagnosing Renee's condition as appendicitis. According to Dr. Mills, Renee could have been operated on right up to 10:00 a.m. on the morning of her death.

Richard and Margaret buried their faces in their hands and wept.

Dr. Mills agreed with Dr. Patterson that Dr. Pickup's working conditions

131

were intolerable and admonished the responsible authorities for allowing such a situation to develop. "The College should look carefully into the standard of medical care here and its equivalent of the provincial nursing body should make recommendations for improving the quality of care and nursing standards," Dr. Mills testified. "Nurses have a responsibility to think first of patient care, and if criticizing the medical profession keeps standards acceptable, then so be it."

Drs. Mills and Patterson both recommended that a pool of doctors be established in rural areas to relieve each other and to allow individual doctors time to upgrade their skills and to take necessary and frequent holidays. No one, Dr. Mills pointed out, should be forced to work alone for prolonged periods of time as Dr. Pickup had been.

"Professional people, lawyers, journalists, accountants, as well as doctors and nurses have difficulty obtaining adequate medical advice for their problems—problems arising from operating solo and being steeped in work. In the case of the medical profession they become physically and emotionally ill, thus affecting their everyday clinical acumen," Dr. Mills testified.

Dr. Patterson suggested that an association be formed on northern Vancouver Island to organize and co-ordinate such a medical pool. Perhaps the association could be called the Renee Smith Foundation, he mused.

Next a Registered Nurse who had worked at St. George's for seven months, until February 1979, was called to the stand after having flown in from Prince Rupert where she was now working. Heather George had been on day shift on January 22nd. "I told Dr. Pickup earlier that day that Renee's condition was deteriorating. He didn't say anything for a few moments. He asked me what I thought. I told him I felt she had a generalized infection from all the things that were happening to her," she testified.

Nurse George had completed her shift and returned to her room in the nurse's residence. She didn't know what had transpired during the four hours between 6:00 p.m. when she had gone off duty and 10:00 p.m. when she received a phone call telling her that Renee was near death. She returned to the hospital and found Dr. Pickup at the nurses' station. "I was surprised he was not in the child's room as she was dying," Nurse George testified. "I think he was physically worn out. I would say he was in a state of shock. He was trying to do his best....I asked him what he was going to do....he told me to administer the sodium cortez [cortisone]...I wanted to give more than he was going to give. He said it was no use, the girl was dying."

Two days before Renee's death Nurse George and Dr. Pickup had worked for sixteen hours on a patient who had gone into cardiac arrest several times. "In that case I had to suggest to Dr. Pickup which drugs I thought he should use, and I don't feel I should have had to do this....When I arrived at the hospital on January 22nd Dr. Pickup seemed to be completely exhausted and somewhat confused," she said.

132

Nurse George stated that she had resigned from St. George's after Renee's death. She cited emotional and physical stress and the hospital's lack of response to three formal, written complaints she had made to the administration regarding irregularities in the doctor's practice and in hospital procedures in general. "I decided to resign after being hospitalized myself. I just decided I had had enough. I felt I couldn't cope any longer," she said. She added that she was having personal problems as well.

Coroner McDonald disallowed detailed discussion of Nurse George's other complaints. "I'm not investigating the hospital, but only the death of Renee Smith," he said. "But maybe we may have to look at the whole forest to find one tree."

By now the inquest had gone on for more than seven days, longer than anyone had expected it to, and Coroner McDonald had approved subpoenas for a total of thirty-eight witnesses, including more nurses, the hospital administration, and Vera Robinson, who had yet to testify. Michael Rhodes had a commitment to appear in the Supreme Court the following Monday, so when the inquest adjourned for the weekend on Friday, June 1st, the Nimpkish Band Council contacted Harry Rankin to ask if he would represent the Smith family for the remainder of the inquest. Rankin agreed, and he and his wife, Johnny, flew up to Alert Bay by chartered plane the following day. Although by now most of the evidence was in, and the direction in which the scales were tipping was quite obvious, the arrival of the tough-talking, famous Harry Rankin made an "Indian victory" seem inevitable.

Going down the road since the inquest began had been like walking a tightrope. When the Rankins arrived and were driven slowly down the road in one of the Band Councillor's shiny new, silver-coloured cars, the whole town was buzzing. People stopped and pointed and stared. Some smirked triumphantly. Others looked frightened.

The first person the Rankins wanted to see was their old friend Gilbert Popovich, mayor of the municipality. Arriving at the mayor's house, everyone smiled awkwardly and Mr. Popovich said he hoped this mess would be straightened out soon so that both ends of town could begin to work together to insure better health care for all residents.

"That makes sense to me," Rankin nodded.

There are a lot of things that can be said about Harry Rankin, and at one time or another somebody has probably said every one of them. But there is one point few people dispute: it's hard to find a match for Harry Rankin fighting in a courtroom. Up to now, the opposing lawyers had done their best to try to humiliate the lawyers working for the "Indian side," and Coroner McDonald had not hesitated to chastise Rhodes for badgering witnesses, or Naknakin for pausing nervously during his cross-examinations. Now, they all smiled ingratiatingly and asked Mr. Rankin, their "esteemed colleague," if arrangements, schedules and seating plans were to his liking. The witnesses seemed to tremble as they took their oaths.

The first person to take the stand after Rankin took over was the Registered Nurse who had been in charge on the night Renee died. It was she who had phoned Dr. Pickup and described Renee as being "ill, restless and uncomfortable" the first time Richard had called her into Renee's room that night. When Dr. Pickup came to the hospital about two hours later, he asked her what was wrong with Renee.

Yes. This did surprise her, she admitted, given that she had spoken to him only a couple of hours earlier.

No, the doctor was not "into his cups," as Mr. Rankin suggested.

Yes, it was unusual that there was no diagnosis.

Yes, charting had been irregular.

No, she didn't know why fluid balance sheets had not been totalled.

"Is there no co-ordination between nurses in the treatment of patients at St. George's?" Rankin demanded.

"Sometimes it is very poor," the nurse replied in a barely audible whisper.

"It was very poor on this day!" Rankin snapped.

A Licensed Practical Nurse testified next. Responding to Rankin's relentless grilling, she said that what had happened to Renee was a result of bad teamwork, poor procedures and a lack of communication among staff. She had noticed that Renee's condition was deteriorating on the night of her death but "it's not my job to call the doctor....It appeared that three nurses were making decisions in the absence of the doctor," the L.P.N. admitted tearfully.

"For Christ's sake, Harry!" Johnny Rankin, seated in the audience behind the lawyer's table, leaned over and scolded her husband in a loud whisper. "They're just working-class girls. You don't have to be so vicious!"

"Well, they're on the wrong God-damned side on this one," Harry growled back over his shoulder, and continued his interrogation.

The federal Indian Health Nurse, Vera Robinson, spent four hours on the stand detailing incorrect nursing procedures she had observed at St. George's. She said that Renee's hospital charts "should be sent to every nursing institution in the country as an example of how not to keep such documents."

"If I had been on duty while Renee was a patient, I would have questioned everything Dr. Pickup did....Each member of a hospital team must be prepared to accept responsibility....this is essential in looking after a patient's welfare," Vera continued. Coroner McDonald stopped her, however, when she began to list her recommendations for improving the situation. He told her she was vindictive and unprofessional and disqualified her as a witness.

The eleventh and final day the inquest heard testimony from the hospital administrator and the Director of Nursing. The administrator admitted having spoken to Dr. Pickup privately about his drinking and having also discussed the matter with the Chairman of the Hospital Board, Reverend Len Perry. The administrator agreed that Dr. Pickup's drinking affected his work and that the doctor consistently refused to comply with requests to prepare patient histories. "I've had complaints, many complaints. We've met with him but he has failed to respond to our requests. We didn't discipline him because he's the only doctor we have," the administrator testified.

The press later questioned him about other matters relating to the administration of the hospital. Was it true that the local coroner's wife was also the medical records librarian and that she and her husband had been close personal friends of the doctor and his wife for many years?

Yes, this was true but she had been hired on the basis of her ability.

Was it true that the hospital purchased food and other supplies from the local merchants?

Well, not always. Purchases were also made from outlets on Vancouver Island.

Was it true that these merchants and/or their wives were often on the hospital's Board of Trustees?

Yes, some of them.

Was it true that local tradesmen were always hired to do necessary repairs, installations, etc. in the hospital and that these men and/or their wives were also frequently members of the hospital's Board of Trustees?

Yes. But in a small town like this, such an overlap is impossible to avoid.

Was it true that there was racial discrimination in St. George's hiring practices?

No, absolutely not. 20 per cent of the staff are Indians. They work in the kitchen and in cleaning. They would be hired in other positions if they applied and were qualified.

The administrator resigned his position shortly after the inquest and left Alert Bay a few months later.

The Nursing Director testified that she had made frequent complaints to both the doctor and to the administrator about the absence of patient histories. "Dr. Pickup has never made any progress notes on patients since I arrived six years ago. It prevents you from doing your duty properly. It prevents the whole hospital from functioning properly." She confirmed that nursing practices were often lax.

The Nursing Director resigned her position shortly after the inquest and left Alert Bay a few months later.

On June 6, 1979 the jury reached their verdict.

We the Jury, find that Renee Bernice Smith, age 11, of P.O. Box 121, Alert Bay, British Columbia, who was certified dead at St. George's Hospital in Alert Bay, B.C. at 2302 hours on the 22nd day of January, 1979, came to her death as a result of severe generalized peritonitis, ruptured appendix and acute gangrenous appendicitis due to the negligence on the part of Dr. Pickup to apply adequate medical care and procedures.

> We, the Jury, conclude this death to be natural and classify it as accidental due to negligence.

Margaret, having maintained her composure throughout the eleven gruelling days of hearings, burst into uncontrolled sobs. Friends and relatives rushed to embrace both her and Richard. Several of the jurors tried unsuccessfully to hold back tears. Reporters, themselves visibly moved by the scene, clamoured for statements.

"It's been very hard on all of us," Richard told the press. "But it was worth it. We don't want what happened to our daughter to ever happen to anyone else again. Indian or White."

The jury foreman went on to read the jury's recommendations.

> We, the Jury, recommend that an investigation by the B.C. Ministry of Health & Welfare, and the B.C. College of Physicians and Surgeons, be held to look into the medical practices of Dr. Pickup and the general standards of medical services in Alert Bay.
>
> Furthermore, we recommend that the appropriate B.C. Nursing Association inquire into nursing care at St. George's Hospital and make recommendations for its improvement.
>
> We, the Jury, feel that the following areas are of special concern and should be given consideration by the investigating bodies.
>
> (1) The College of Physicians and Surgeons and the St. George's Hospital Board should make every effort to get another practicing doctor immediately.
>
> (2) Oral communication between patient-nurse-doctor and administrating body be improved.
>
> (3) When minors are involved, guardian or parent should be fully informed of all circumstances.
>
> (4) That the Consent to Operation and Treatment form be redesigned to clarify the difference between medical or surgical treatment. Also some onus be placed on person(s) signing as witnesses, on these forms. For example, they could be asked to sign a statement, e.g. I hearby certify that I have fully explained the above form to person signing.
>
> (5) That a more reliable and faster means of getting X-Ray and test results to and from hospital, laboratory and specialists (such as private courier service versus postal service) be found.
>
> (6) To alleviate the existence of a sole practitioner covering an area for an extended period of time.
>
> (7) It is felt that Exhibits 22, 23, 24 [copies of Renee's hospital and medical records, Drs. Mills' and Patterson's recommendations for medical services to rural areas] of this inquest be distributed to all investigating bodies, for their consideration, with our strong recommendation for implementation.

(8) Stricter enforcement of the hospital rules and regulations governing the medical staff of St. George's Hospital, Alert Bay, B.C.
(9) We strongly recommend that the people of Alert Bay get involved
in the administration of St. George's Hospital.

On the other side of the room, mouths tightly closed, hands clenched and
backs held rigidly straight, Dr. Pickup's supporters rose silently and left the
hall. Dr. Pickup refused to speak to the press but close friends of his were
quoted as saying they expected he would resign and take a well-earned rest.
Mayor Popovich said he would seek assistance from the regional board to
have another doctor located in town immediately. "I feel we've all let Pickup
down. I do not blame him entirely. If we have a second-class system, I think
the Municipal Council is to blame. Maybe we should have taken an interest
in it....But a majority of the blame lies with the College. They knew God-
damned well that this area didn't have enough medical staff. It's fine to say
another doctor is needed here, but the cold hard facts are that doctors don't
want to come to Alert Bay."

Vera Robinson agreed. "Pickup has been let down by people who love, respect
and honour him for what he has done in the past. He is a lonely man. The
system failed him."

Later that evening a party was organized at the Legion for Dr. Pickup.

Going down the road after the verdict was announced took on the
characteristics of a victory parade, for a while. Everyone had their own way
of acknowledging this victory, from outright and somewhat vengeful celebration; to bold-faced smirking, smiling and sarcasm at the cash registers manned
by local businessmen; to angry and sometimes drunken outpourings of years
of repressed bitterness; to quiet satisfaction marked by heads held slightly higher
and gazes met more directly; to gracious forgiveness.

There were few historical precedents for what had happened. The tables had
indeed been turned when the pillars of the White community stood exposed
to the world, by a legal forum, as having alcohol problems, or questionable
professional ethics, or debatable administrative competence. Their integrity
was suspect and negligence had caused the death of a child.

Indians may have "won," but the price paid—a child's life, a family's ordeal,
and the public exposure of two insular communities—was high for all concerned.

NOTES:

Sources for this chapter are: personal notes, tape recordings, interviews with participants
and observers, newspaper reports, personal notes, and Gottschau, W.(ed) (1979), *Inquest
Into the Death of Renee Bernice Smith Held at the Alert Bay Coroner's Court*, April
18th and 19th, 1979, Transcript of Proceedings, Vols. I & II. All statements enclosed
by quotation marks are verbatim quotes and are part of the public record and derived
from either newspaper reports or official court transcripts. Mr. Bill Smith, of the *Victoria*

Daily Colonist, provided the most thorough press coverage. Statements attributed to people and/or groups which are not enclosed in quotation marks are reconstructions from my personal notes and are not necessarily verbatim quotes. Original sources have been edited for logical sequencing, consistency and ease of reading.

[1]Rozovsky, Lorne E. "The Patient's Duty to Himself," *DIMENSIONS in Health Services*, December, 1979, pp. 27-28.

[2]British Columbia Medical Association (BCMA) *Federal/Provincial Indian Health Committee Report* (1974), Dr. H. J. Pickup, Corresponding Member.

[3]Ibid.

[4]Ibid.

[5]Ibid.

[6]*The Canadian Nurse*, October, 1978, Vol. 74, p. 40.

[7]*History of Alert Bay and District*, op. cit., p. 24.

[8]Ibid., pp. 13, 24.

CHAPTER 6

A Symbolic Victory

In response to the announcement of the jury's verdict, the Attorney-General for B.C., Garde Gardom, told the press that prosecution of Dr. Pickup was "obviously a consideration." His office would review the jury's findings and the transcript of the Inquest before taking any action. They awaited receipt of these documents.

The Minister of Health for B.C., Robert McClelland, said that it was up to the College of Physicians and Surgeons and not him to decide whether or not Dr. Pickup should resign, but he "assumed the doctor would take whatever action he felt was necessary." In the meantime, he appointed Dr. Charles Ballam, senior medical consultant for the provincial Ministry of Health, to chair a Board of Inquiry. McClelland hastened to add that Pickup's negligence was an isolated case and not indicative of the state of health care in small communities throughout the province.

The Registered Nurses Association of B.C. (RNABC) released a letter they had written to the B.C. Ministry of Health to the press. It read:

RNABC has watched with concern the inquest into events at St. George's Hospital, Alert Bay. Our ability to take action in this matter has been limited by two factors: 1. The fact that nearly all the nurses involved are not registered. As you know, RNABC has no jurisdiction over un-registered graduate nurses who may practice in B.C. 2. Lack of access to official documentation.

With the inquest verdict delivered, it is clear that your ministry is likely to conduct further investigations. RNABC offers its services to your ministry during those investigations....

The Deputy Registrar of the B.C. College of Physicians and Surgeons, Dr. Craig Arnold, announced that they would hold an internal inquiry into Dr. Pickup's competence and that the jury's recommendations would "receive serious consideration."

People in the Indian community continued their campaign. The Nimpkish Band Council wrote to all the responsible authorities asking for a second doctor for the island immediately. Letters, affidavits and transcripts of interviews about experiences with local health services were collected. People were encouraged to take out the one-dollar annual membership in the St. George's Hospital Society which would enable them to vote at society meetings and participate in gaining some control over St. George's.

On June 12, 1979, six days after the inquest adjourned, the St. George's Hospital Society held a special meeting. The Nimpkish Indian Band sent a delegation of newly signed-up members to the meeting to present the following special resolution:

(1) THAT Dr. Pickup's hospital privileges at St. George's Hospital be suspended.

(2) THAT the administration of St. George's show more responsibility by guaranteeing the following:

(a) THAT properly trained nurses and technicians with a high degree of professional ethics be hired.

(b) THAT an alcohol rehabilitation program be implemented at St. George's Hospital.

(c) THAT at least TWO competent doctors [be available] at all times.

(d) THAT an Advisory Board made up of elected or appointed representatives from bands served by St. George's Hospital [be established] to oversee services to Native people.

The Chairman of the Hospital Board announced that they had been advised by legal counsel that they could not suspend Dr. Pickup's privileges on the basis of the jury's verdict but would have to wait until the College of Physicians and Surgeons, the body mandated by the legislature to discipline and license doctors, had released the results of their inquiry.[1]

The St. George's Hospital Board concluded that Dr. Pickup would continue to practise but that they, and the College, were doing their very best to get a second doctor to come to Alert Bay. This task was being made more difficult by the climate of confrontation which existed in the community and it was incumbent upon all to pull together and offset the bad publicity the town had received.

140

The band delegation objected. How could patients, and particularly Native patients, be expected to continue to see Dr. Pickup and be treated at St. George's, after the evidence that had come out at the Inquest? The Chairman ruled the band's representative out of order. According to the St. George's Hospital Society's Rules of Order, the band's motion had not been properly submitted in advance of the meeting. The Native delegation walked out.

On the afternoon of that day, the Nimpkish Band Council composed a telegram which stated that the Village needed a second doctor *immediately*, that Dr. Pickup was continuing to practise and the Hospital Board was not prepared to do anything about this or any of the other recommendations made by the inquest's jury. They demanded that Pickup's license be revoked immediately and that the provincial government suspend the Hospital Board and appoint a trustee to oversee the operation of the hospital until the public inquiry was held. Telegrams were sent to the College of Physicians and Surgeons, the B.C. Ministry of Health, the B.C. Ministry of the Attorney-General, the Registered Nurses Association of B.C., the Minister of Indian and Northern Affairs, the Minister of National Health and Welfare, the Regional Director of Medical Services for the Indian Health Division, the Union of British Columbia Indian Chiefs, the United Native Nations, the Native Brotherhood of British Columbia and the National Indian Brotherhood. The Indian organizations immediately sent telegrams supporting the Band's demands to all the responsible authorities.

Individuals wrote letters to the Hospital Board protesting their decision, including the following one which came from a non-Indian couple in Sointula:

> We are disappointed with your decision which in effect gives support to incompetence as found by the recent inquest into the death of Renee Smith. We fear that if you do not make a decision to take strong corrective measures that solutions will be found by simply eliminating St. George's.
>
> Dr. Pickup has built up a large following over his 30 years in the North Island. We attribute this large following to the 'do-it-yourself' medical practice prevalently found here. People can pick up the phone and get prescribed an amazing array of medications that ordinarily would require thorough medical examination. Probably most people suspect that this practice would cease with new practitioners at St. George's.
>
> It is not easy for people to write letters being critical of a man that so many people believe in. It is akin to criticizing other peoples religious practices. The Nimpkish Band has taken on a formidable task in championing medical reform for the people of the North Island.
>
> We feel guilty for not having sought out effective avenues of complaint against medical practices we know to be careless at worst and primitive at best. We feel guilty when years ago our neighbor, G.T.,

died. We said nothing where it might have counted. Again when Louisa James died, we said nothing.

We have actually heard the argument that Dr. Pickup should be retained because he works hard. We think this is fallacious reasoning to suggest that good medical practice will follow the number of hours worked and the dedication of an elderly practitioner with a publicly documented drinking problem.

It is our opinion that in seeking another doctor on the staff, you will not find one as long as Dr. Pickup is allowed to have hospital privileges at St. George's. We have seen recently how doctors will not testify against each other and we would suspect they would show great reluctance to put themselves in a position to view incompetent medical practice on a daily basis.

We wish to emphasize that we think the people responsible for the death of Renee Smith are those like ourselves, who realize the incompetence of Dr. Pickup and said nothing; not those of you who truly believe he is a good doctor.

Even some local teachers were moved to take a stand:

We, the undersigned, teachers in the community of Alert Bay, wish to express our support for a full scale Public Inquiry into the medical care available to this community as proposed by the Nimpkish Band and Kwakewlth District Council and concerned citizens.

Some of us have been teachers in this community for several years and have witnessed questionable practices concerning the medical care of our students.

It is essential that the health needs of each individual child be foremost in the minds of those of us who attend to them.

Because of this concern, we, the undersigned, insist the Inquiry be a thorough and just investigation, that encompasses all aspects of medical care.

This, then, was another significant turning point. The possibility of a resolution being arrived at locally no longer existed. Dr. Pickup and the Hospital Board were clearly impervious to informal sanctions like gossip and public shame, and inquest juries' verdicts carry no powers of enforcement. The band, having exhausted these channels and being unable, still, to have any of their demands met at a local level, began a process of public lobbying of both provincial and federal government ministries, with the support of Indian political organizations, to establish a public inquiry into health care. The arena had been expanded once again to include the federal government—at the *federal*, rather than regional, level; organized allies, rather than simply "public sympathy," were sought; the Nimpkish Band Council was now in charge, rather than an amorphous grouping of Renee's relatives and "concerned citizens." And, the definition of the problem now clearly included both Dr. Pickup's drinking, the administration of the hospital, and "Indian health" in general.

Tension in town mounted and the press began to question people about the potential for violence to erupt. "You've got rednecks in both communities, but no guns will be drawn by this side," Chief Roy Cranmer assured them.

Meanwhile, local men with boats or fishing jobs—fewer this year than last, as there had been fewer last year than the year before—got ready for the salmon season. Renee's family prepared a memorial potlatch in her honour, and the Indian community prepared for the annual June Sports Days held every year.

Begun in 1958 by the Village's Cormorant Athletic Association, "June Sports"—or "Indian Sports"—is a significant event in the life of the Indian community. June Sports begins the fishing season, as the men usually leave for the west coast of Vancouver Island or the north coast after June Sports, and few of the village children return to school after the weekend. There is a road parade with floats and marchers, and a boat parade out on the water with fishing boats decorated by banners and streamers. The Anglican Minister blesses the fishing fleet, and the soccer tournament begins. Games are played all weekend, including "Old Ladies" and "Old Mens" games in which everyone from about 20 up who isn't a serious soccer player participates, and kids' sports like three-legged races and watermelon-eating contests. The weekend winds up with a big dance after the final, championship game. Indian soccer teams from all over the coast, the lower mainland and Vancouver Island come to play. Most of the trophies awarded in the seemingly endless list of eligible categories are donated by local families in memory of deceased relatives, or in honour of individuals who have donated time, money and moral support to the teams over the years. Many are hand-carved replicas of totem poles made by local artists.

June Sports is the weekend when "everyone comes home." Old friendships and love affairs are rekindled, new ones begun; old feuds and enmities are resolved or revived and new ones begun; and long-gone relatives are brought back into the fold.

St. George's Hospital and June Sports have a very special connection. Chief James Sewid described the origins of this relationship in his autobiography. Recalling his experiences as the first Indian appointed to St. George's fund-raising committee in the '50s, Chief Sewid says:

> I thought a lot about what we could do to raise money for the hospital and it just came to me that it would be a good idea to bring the potlatch custom and the dancing out to the surface again and let the public see it....
> The first thing I did was go and talk to one of the leading men of

the people. All the old people were still alive then and we wrote a letter to all the chiefs of the different tribes....So when they came I called a meeting for all the chiefs in the community hall. There were a lot of them, about ten or fifteen of the leading men of each village....I said 'I think it is a worthy cause to bring you here and we can all support St. George's Hospital because we all use it.'

That night the hall was really crowded with people from all over the area....We must have had a five-hour do there that night and I think it was one of the biggest dances because all the big chiefs were there, the prominent and noble men of all the villages.[2]

June Sports incorporated these public fund-raising dances, and since the revised Indian Act of 1951 had omitted the clauses banning potlatching, such dances were gradually replaced by potlatches and June Sports also came to be the time when these were held. Money raised at the soccer tournaments continued to be donated to St. George's Hospital for the purchase of new equipment, specifically X-ray equipment, due to the continued high incidence of T.B. and other respiratory ailments among the Indian population.

June Sports also serves as an annual measure of the mood of the Village. When things are not good within the host community it shows up at June Sports. Few people bother to volunteer to work on the organization of the festivities, fewer "migrants" than usual make the trip home, not many teams are invited, and big fights occur among the fans over the soccer games. June Sports had been marred in recent years by the drinking deaths of two young men.

This year, 1979, the June Sports Committee had decided that the parade's theme should be the United Nations International Year of the Child. The planning committee was huge.

The parade was led by a large truck festooned with broom and lilac and a huge wreath with a banner bearing the words IN LOVING MEMORY OF RENEE SMITH. Other cars and floats followed, each one decorated to illustrate one of the ten principles of the United Nations Declaration of the Rights of the Child.

A pick-up truck carrying children dressed in different national costumes carried the banner reading: EVERY CHILD SHALL ENJOY THESE RIGHTS REGARDLESS OF RACE, COLOR, SEX, LANGUAGE, RELIGION OR POLITICAL OPINION.

EVERY CHILD SHALL BE ENTITLED TO A NAME AND NATIONALITY proclaimed the Land Claims Committee car. Cars and bicycles followed, carrying more signs, balloons and streamers: EVERY CHILD HAS A RIGHT TO PROPER NUTRITION; EVERY CHILD HAS A RIGHT TO EDUCATION; EVERY CHILD HAS A RIGHT TO BE LOVED.

The largest and most graphic float was the band's flatbed truck on which were strewn bedridden, bandaged, ketchup-bloodied children moaning, groaning and crying out with great enthusiasm. The giant banner on the truck read EVERY CHILD HAS A RIGHT TO ADEQUATE MEDICAL CARE.

The parade took its usual route. Beginning at St. George's Hospital it wound its way down the main road, through the tiny business district and up the hill, less than a mile away, to the soccer field on the reserve. Spectators along the route cheered and waved. A few raised clenched fists. Some glared angrily. Others looked away, embarrassed. Things had changed somewhat since Chief Sewid had proudly taken his place on the hospital committee, but who could argue with the United Nations?

The following week the Nimpkish Band Council and its staff drew up a list of objectives for the promised public inquiry. They were:

(1) to prevent Dr. Pickup from practising medicine.

(2) to re-organize St. George's to insure that it meets the needs of the community. Suggestions for re-organization:

(a) properly trained nurses and technicians with a high degree of professional ethics [be hired].

(b) [institute] an alcohol rehabilitation program—an effective one

(c) at least two competent doctors [be available] at all times

(d) establishment of an advisory board made up of elected or appointed representatives from all bands served by St. George's to oversee services to Native people

(e) preventative and educational services.

(3) To expose to the Canadian public the situation as it has existed for so many years and to determine the factors that have contributed to this and to determine the public accountability of the following organizations:

(a) B.C. College of Physicians and Surgeons

(b) St. George's Hospital Board

(c) Registered Nurses Association of B.C.

(d) B.C. Medical Association

(e) B.C. Hospitals Association

(f) Federal Government Indian Health Services

(g) Province of B.C. Health Department

(4) To encourage other Native peoples with similar problems to speak out and to demand better services

(5) To show the public the need to oppose federal government cut-backs in Indian health services.

(6) If at all possible, to obtain compensation for people who have been disabled due to incompetence on the part of Dr. Pickup and/or any of the organizations listed in #3.

We told the press we wanted answers to these questions: We want to know why did St. George's Hospital board allow Dr. Pickup continued privileges at the hospital during the years of complaints about inadequate care and excessive drinking? Why have other doctors who've corrected Dr. Pickup's mistakes not taken action? Why hasn't the Government found a way to ensure that remote areas have more than one doctor? Why doesn't the College investigate the competence of doctors? And why don't nurses receive special training for work in remote areas with Indians?

In hindsight, of course, it is obvious that objective number 3 would have required something akin to several Royal Commissions and objective number 6 would have involved years of civil litigation. However, this is evidence of the magnitude of the victory achieved at the inquest, as it appeared to those whose focus was political relations on Cormorant Island. Nothing seemed unattainable to the local activists at this point. Had all their charges, and then some, not been validated beyond any reasonable doubt by testimony at the inquest?

NOTES:

[1]The *Canadian Medical Association Journal* of October 6, 1979, Vol. 121, p. 970 had the following to say about this point.

> Physicians, generally, over the years, have supported the concept that hospital staff membership is a privilege and that the extent of the privileges granted should be recommended to the hospital board by the medical staff advisory committee or its equivalent, and should be dependent upon the training and competence of those applying. Those physicians who have been denied privileges or who have had their privileges reduced have access to the courts. The courts almost without exception have supported the right of hospital boards to grant or deny privileges...

[2]Spradley, James P. (1972) (ed) *Guests Never Leave Hungry: The Autobiography of James Sewid, A Kwakiutl Indian*, Kingston: McGill-Queens University Press, pp. 158-160.

CHAPTER 7

I Cannot Hear What You Are Saying Because I Can See What You Are: "Indian Health"

I. THERE ARE NONE SO BLIND AS THOSE WHO WILL NOT SEE

There is no question native Indians should have the right to determine their health care needs and how they can be met most appropriately. But...native peoples should make these decisions within the established democratic process of this country and within the context of one comprehensive health care system.
—Robert H. McClelland, Minister of Health for British Columbia,
"Statement on Indian Health Care in B.C.,"
November, 1979

During the five weeks of the inquest's adjournment, from April 19th to May 28th, individuals in the community and the Nimpkish Band Council had continued to write to the B.C. College of Physicians and Surgeons, the federal Indian Health Division and the B.C. Ministry of Health, requesting that a permanent second doctor be stationed at Alert Bay and re-asserting the demand that a full-scale, public inquiry be established into the entire health care delivery system in the Kwakwaka'wakw area. The provincial Ministry of Health had

responded by appointing a seven-member inquiry panel, including representatives of the B.C. Health Ministry, the College of Physicians and Surgeons,
the B.C. Medical Association, the B.C. Hospitals Association and the Registered
Nurses Association of B.C. The inquiry's chairman, senior medical consultant
Dr. Charles Ballam, promised the hearings would be public. The inquiry could
not be convened, however, until after the inquest's jury returned their verdict,
for fear of prejudicing the outcome of the inquest. The band agreed to these
terms and retained the services of Harry Rankin to represent them whenever
the inquiry got underway.

After the inquest the British Columbia Ministry of Health and Dr. Ballam
elected to consult with the Nimpkish Band through the press and publicly
announced the terms of reference under which the inquiry would operate, without
any prior direct consultation. The band first became aware of the organization
of the Ballam Inquiry when a reporter called and asked for a response to the
following terms of reference.

Meetings would be held in the hospital administrator's office. The band would
be allotted three hours to present its case. There would be no access to medical
records, no right to cross-examination and much of the inquiry was to be held
in camera. Furthermore, the inquiry would begin immediately, despite the band's
request that it be postponed until the fall since many of the men, and almost
all the Band Councillors, were out fishing during the summer months. To add
insult to injury, Dr. Ballam told the press that he was not coming to Alert
Bay in response to the band's petition but rather in response to a request from
the Hospital Board for assistance. His main objective, he said, was to "reconcile
the community" which had been "torn asunder" by recent events. The situation was "too explosive" to wait until the fall. Alert Bay was a "tinder-box."

This theme, i.e. that an otherwise harmonious and united community had
been suddenly divided into warring factions by the events surrounding Renee
Smith's death, was raised repeatedly by both Dr. Pickup's local supporters
and by representatives of the provincial government. Despite repeated statements
by band members to the press, and to anyone else who would listen, that "the
divisions have always been here. They're just showing up now and everyone
is upset because it's us Indians who are complaining about them," this explanation continued to be put forward.

On June 16, 1979, ten days after the inquest's verdict had been announced
and following several unsuccessful attempts to negotiate the terms of reference
for the inquiry with the B.C. Ministry of Health, the Nimpkish Band Council
and the Kwakiutl District Council, representing 3500 Kwakwaka'wakw
people, issued the following press release:

> We refuse to participate in the upcoming inquiry into medical services
> here in Alert Bay as it is set up presently.
>
> Four months ago we petitioned for an Inquest into one death and

a public inquiry into medical services here in general.... Evidence brought out during that inquest shocked us even more—evidence of improper administration and nursing procedures at St. George's Hospital. Among their recommendations the jury asked that an inquiry be held. Our goal remains the same as when we started asking that our problems be looked into, and was best expressed by Renee's father, Richard Smith, when he said, "We do not want what happened to our daughter to happen to anyone else—Indian or White."

Now we are told, third and fourth hand...that the "public" inquiry is to be held in the hospital administrator's office, which could not hold more than 15 people. How can it be public when there is no room for the public? We also hear that our representative will not be permitted to ask questions and that the inquiry board will not even be staying in our community while they are here but will be commuting from Port McNeill.[1]

We have many questions which we want answered and yet we are not to ask questions?

Representatives of the government and the College of Physicians and Surgeons continue to refer to Renee Smith's death as an "isolated incident" even though they have been presented with evidence that it is not "an isolated incident" but rather the inevitable result of the type of medical care Dr. Pickup and St. George's Hospital have been providing our people for quite some time now.

We can only draw from this the conclusion that the death of one Indian child is not important enough for these powerful people to take an honest look at the situation and to do something about it.

We have been receiving substandard medical care, the authorities have been aware of it and have allowed it to continue and we are determined to change this situation. We are entitled to proper medical care like all other citizens of Canada and we intend to guarantee that we receive it.

Our children are no less precious than the Minister of Health's and the members of the College of Physicians and Surgeons...

We are requesting an immediate meeting with the provincial Minister of Health and the Federal Minister of National Health and Welfare.

In order to insure that a truly *public* inquiry is held, we demand the following:

(1) That a meeting place large enough to accommodate the public be found.

(2) That all parties concerned agree upon an impartial chairperson.

(3) That no closed meetings be held with any group or individual. Means can be found to protect any confidentiality necessary.

(4) Cross-examination of witnesses be permitted.

(5) All records be made available: Dr. Pickup's office; billing records; St. George's Hospital; Federal Indian Health Dept.

(6) That all parties concerned be given the opportunity to study the evidence brought forward at the Renee Smith inquest.

Since meeting the above conditions would take time we suggest a postponement to a mutually agreeable time and that the following interim measures be taken to assure our people proper medical care in the interim until an inquiry can arrive at a permanent resolution of our problems.

(1) Dr. Pickup's license to practise be suspended until the inquiry.

(2) St. George's Hospital Board be dissolved and the hospital placed under trusteeship until such time as a proper inquiry can be held.

(3) The B.C. College of Physicians and Surgeons, the Department of Indian Affairs, the Department of National Health and Welfare and the provincial Ministry of Health join forces to insure that two competent doctors are sent to serve our medical needs immediately.

Dr. Ballam agreed to meet one of these demands. He said he would start looking for a larger room in which to hold his inquiry.

Support for the band's criticism of the Ballam Inquiry came from the unlikely source of Coroner McDonald, who took the unusual step of contacting the press himself. "My jury called for an Inquiry. They meant an inquiry with a big 'I'. I hope we didn't spend eleven days probing this girl's death in vain," he said. McDonald told reporters that his interpretation of his jury's recommendation was that a full-scale inquiry would be held under the Public Inquiries Act, with a judge as chairman.

By June 21st the Nimpkish Band's staff had prepared a package containing copies of all petitions; a summation of the main points of evidence given at the inquest; a copy of the jury's verdict and recommendations; and summaries of the thirty-three letters, affidavits and transcripts of interviews setting out complaints about Dr. Pickup and the hospital staff, twenty-seven from Indians, six from non-Indians, including two registered nurses who had worked at the hospital recently (See Chapter 3). These packages were sent to the College of Physicians and Surgeons, the B.C. Ministry of Health, the B.C. Ministry of the Attorney-General; the Registered Nurses Association of B.C., the Minister of Indian and Northern Affairs, the Minister of National Health and Welfare, the Regional Director of Medical Services, the Union of British Columbia Indian Chiefs, the United Native Nations, the Native Brotherhood of British Columbia and the National Indian Brotherhood. The Indian organizations again immediately sent telegrams supporting the band's demands to all the responsible authorities.

Undaunted by the band's refusal to participate, Dr. Ballam and his crew ploughed ahead with their inquiry. They did agree to meet with the Nimpkish

Band Council, once, informally, to listen to their complaints about Dr. Pickup and the hospital, and the structure of the Ballam Inquiry.

Arriving at the old residential school, St. Michael's, which now housed the band administration offices and the band clinic, the nattily dressed, well-groomed members of Dr. Ballam's team reclined on chairs, cupped their chins in their hands and cast sidelong glances at each other. The Band Councillors, most of whom had run up from the docks and their boats to attend the meeting, and who smelled indisputably fishy in their scaly rubber boots, plaid "Mac" jackets and baseball caps, filed in. The Band Manager began the meeting with a summary of events to date: the background of years of complaints, the evidence brought out at the inquest, the refusal of the Hospital Board to revoke Dr. Pickup's privileges or to discuss the Native community's proposals for restructuring the hospital administration, the need for a thorough, and truly public, inquiry. Dr. Ballam, the province's senior medical consultant, announced that he and his colleagues were prepared to listen to all the band's "real *or imagined*" complaints. This was too much for one of the Councillors who exploded:

Goddam it you guys! If there's one thing we goddam know about it's drinkin'! Can't you even give us that?

Like, say I've got a man on my boat and say—like we all drink eh? What the hell... —but let's say this guy gets into the sauce pretty heavy like and he's drinkin' on the job too. Well, let's say he's an older man, eh? A good man, put in a lot of years. Maybe he's my uncle or something like that. Well, I'll probably carry him. And the rest of the boys, they'll probably feel the same way, like they won't mind carrying him for a while, 'cause...like we all get old eh? Now let's say one day he's snapped up and he lets go the line and the beachman gets killed. Well, hey, that's it eh? Can't carry him any longer. Most men I know would get off the boat themselves. They'd have enough whatever to quit before someone has to tell them to. Like they'd know what they'd done and maybe this beachman he's a young guy with a few kids, and the boozer, well he's going to have to live with that...what he done.

Now maybe there's people who would say that I should've gotten rid of the old man a lot sooner. Like, I'm the skipper and I should've known that something like this was goin' to happen and maybe it was my responsibility to tell the old guy to get off. Well, I don't know. That's a tough one. 'Cause like I said, you wanna give a guy a break. Don't wanna dump him as soon as he's got problems. But then again, maybe they're right when they say, well I got to worry about the other guys on the boat too.

We know about that one...I mean...we understand that...it's tough...

But, hey! I don't fix it so he can go work on that white guys' boat over there and put them in danger instead!

151

A few individuals from the band did appear before the Ballam Inquiry despite the Band Council's official refusal to participate. The Zone Director for federal Indian Health/Medical Services, Dr. Mary Habgood, testified about local health conditions. "Alcoholism is a plague on the reserve," Dr. Habgood warned. "Children have difficulty growing mentally, emotionally and physically." Her testimony was among the few that were public, and was reported at length in the press.

Chief Roy Cranmer was asked by reporters to respond. "It's not exactly what we had in mind," he said.

The Ballam Inquiry board issued its report and recommendations on July 21, 1979. They proposed the following changes:

(1) That a revision of the Society Constitution and By-Laws be done to insure greater Native participation in the hospital society.

(2) That a temporary administrator be appointed as an interim measure.

(3) That minutes be kept of all Hospital Board meetings.

(4) That staff vacancies be advertised and that all candidates, native and non-native, have equal employment opportunity.

(5) That the hiring of immediate relatives of senior hospital staff be prohibited.

(6) That the hospital seek Canadian Hospital Association accreditation.

(7) That the scope of surgery performed be limited.

(8) That to deal with medical staffing, surgical limitation, obstetrics, referral-out policies, etc. the hospital seeks assistance from the B.C.M.A., the College and the B.C. Ministry of Health.

(9) That formal liaison be established with the Port McNeill Hospital Board and the Port Hardy Hospital Board.

In all, the Ballam Inquiry board listed 28 recommendations for improving hospital procedures, including the review of all doctors' standing orders, the reduction and clarification of the nursing staff's discretionary authority, standardization of record-keeping and the maintenance of patient histories, and the development of more efficient reporting and communication among staff members. The panel raised the possibility of changing the hospital's name to one which "might less amplify the dominance of the non-native population as exemplified in the present name," and the development of special evaluation procedures to assist Hospital Boards in small communities to evaluate complaints regarding staff drug, alcohol, mental problems "or other aberration attributed to or alleged of Medical staff where the information is less than would be required to lay formal complaint."

No explicit mention was made of Dr. Pickup in the Ballam Report. The inquiry panel did not, however, ignore the needs of the Native population. They recommended that detox services be established in consultation with "Indian Health Services, the Drug and Alcohol Commission, the Band Council and other involved agencies," and that interpreters be available to Native patients in order to help them to better understand hospital regulations such as limitations on the number of visitors, and the proper way to sign consent forms. Furthermore, it recommended that the Nimpkish Band encourage its young people to pursue medical careers.

Dr. Ballam advised against the holding of a public inquiry for the following reasons:

> (1) It would add to the divisiveness now evident;
>
> (2) It would not necessarily expose the truths having pertinence to improving health care in this area, but would run the almost certain risk of becoming bogged down in claim and counter claim as to be counter-productive and hence, it could delay implementation of needed positive objectives and goals which can be accomplished within the framework recommended...

Finally, they recommended that Reverend Eric Powell, an Anglican missionary who had spent a lot of time in the Kwakwaka'wakw area, and had considerable influence among elderly people in the Indian community, be appointed special consultant to the Minister of Health and interim co-ordinator of the hospital. Reverend Powell's mandate was to "...provide leadership and assistance to the Board of Trustees at St. George's Hospital and the community...." The Social Credit Minister of Health announced beneficently that this would insure that the native Indians in Alert Bay had a voice in the organization of health care in their community.

Once again, press releases were issued and appeals were made to all the Indian organizations for support. This time the band's statement read as follows:

> As to the appointment of Eric Powell as Co-ordinator for the hospital. We are at a loss to understand what his role is to be....What we have here is a medical problem and a political problem...This is not a spiritual problem....Many of our people have a good deal of respect for Reverend Powell and we mean no personal offence whatsoever. We simply fail to see how he can do anything to solve this problem. Apparently the provincial government does not realize that the time has long since passed when Indian peoples' problems can be solved by missionaries—however well-intentioned they may be....
>
> We do not recall ever putting forward any complaints about the hospital's name.

The Hospital Board ratified Dr. Ballam's recommendations on July 31st, 1979.[2]

Reverend Powell accepted the appointment offered him by the provincial government despite the fact that the Native people for whom he was supposed to be the voice did not officially meet with him. Again, while the elected representatives of the Native community, i.e. the Band Council, were not consulted, some individual band members, particularly a few elderly people, did discuss their opinions about the controversy with him and he apparently felt satisfied that he had received input from the Native community.

Reverend Powell's findings were, by now, predictable. He found "the Board, the Administrator, staff and doctor very co-operative and pleasant." The hospital staff, he said, were "competent, professional and maintained a high level of patient care." There was no doubt in his mind that "alcoholism was the major cause for the majority of health care problems on the island." He recommended the establishment of a detox centre at St. George's, and the hiring of a provincial social worker with special training in alcohol treatment who would supervise this program and "...assist, support and provide consultation to native Indian Counsellors (subject to the approval of the Band Council)." Privately he told people he would speak to the Minister about changing the name of the hospital. An Indian name, perhaps, would be more appropriate and would help change the image of the hospital in Indian people's minds.

The Hospital Board did agree, under Reverend Powell's direction, to restructure its Board of Trustees as follows:

(a) 1 person appointed by the Lieutenant Governor in Council;

(b) 1 person appointed annually by the Hospital Board of the Regional Hospital District;

(c) 1 person appointed annually by the members of the Hospital Auxilliary;

(d) 6 persons elected by the members of the Society to be made up as follows:

2 persons resident in the Nimpkish Reserve who are Indians within the meaning of the Indian Act;

2 persons resident in the Municipality of Alert Bay;

1 person resident in the community of Sointula;

1 person resident in any of the Vancouver Island area of the Mount Waddington Regional District.

Again, the Nimpkish Band Council, the Whe-La-La-U Area Council, and the Kwakiutl District Council rejected this "solution." Two positions out of nine on the Board of Trustees would not give the Native representatives any decision-making power, and did not reflect the make-up of the patient population which was over 50 per cent Native. The Board's stipulation that these representatives would have to be *status* Indians[3] resident on the Nimpkish Reserve meant that non-status Indians would be unable to participate, *as Indians*. (A status or non-status Indian individual, resident in the municipality could, of course, be elected to one of the municipality's two positions.) Members of Kwakwa̱ka'wakw bands other than the Nimpkish who lived in the surrounding villages, and residents of the Whe-La-La-U All Bands Reserve, all of which were served by St. George's, would be excluded. None of the bands would be permitted to elect or appoint their own representatives to the Hospital Board in a manner that they considered appropriate.

A weary Band Manager, Pearl Alfred, told the press, "The sad thing about this whole affair is that the Minister and his advisors can see nothing wrong with the attitude they have adopted. It was a clear case of Indians being told 'You be quiet. We know what's best for you.'"

One band member, Gloria Cranmer Webster, wrote personally to Bob McClelland, B. C.'s Minister of Health:

> Mr. Powell's recommendation that, first of all, there should be a detoxification centre is appalling in the context of Renee Smith's death. Renee was not an alcoholic, nor was her death due to her alcoholism, although it might have been due to someone else's alcoholism. There is no guarantee that establishing a detoxification centre in Alert Bay will prevent the needless death of another 11-year-old child.

The Minister replied:

> I cannot stress too often that the opportunity of taking part in the planning and operation of our health facilities is available to you if you will only take those steps which are necessary. Up to this point, however, your people seem to have chosen to take a path which would lead to non-involvement in the affairs of your local health system.
> I continue to have full confidence in Mr. Powell....

The Indian people in Alert Bay who were experienced in trying to communicate with various levels of government were frustrated and disappointed by the provincial government's responses, but they were not shocked. British Columbia's policies regarding Native peoples develop from a fundamental starting position which limits their scope and determines their boundaries: according to the Social Credit government, aboriginal societies, as they are defined by aboriginal people, do not exist.

B.C. Natives have been arguing for more than 100 years that prior to the arrival of Europeans they were the sovereign owners of the land and resources of what is now the province of British Columbia. Since none of these lands or resources have been "ceded, sold, or lost in war," this "aboriginal title," as it is known, persists to the present day. From aboriginal title, the Native position asserts, flows the right to self-determination and self-government. It is the recognition of these rights that they insist must form the basis of their relationship to Canadian society.

The B.C. government's position begins with a denial of these claims. To support their position, the province relies on a legal and political interpretation of history which argues that *if* aboriginal peoples lived in organized societies— rather than in roaming, ungoverned bands of "savages"—and did practise some form of property ownership at the time of initial European colonization, such aboriginal title ceased to exist when B.C. entered Confederation in 1871, at which time all land deemed not to be in private hands became the property of the Crown. From this starting position, the province argues that Native peoples to-day have no distinct relationship to land or resources, and are therefore only one of many ethnic groups within the province, distinguished primarily by their many "problems." It is on this basis that the government of British Columbia refuses to enter into land claims negotiations with B.C. Natives or to recognize their right to self-determination or self-government.

The provincial solution to the "Indian problem" proposes doing away with any legal or political differentiations between Indians and the rest of the population and assimilating Indians into mainstream society. Therefore, the provincial government not only will not negotiate land claims, but they also oppose the special relationship between Native peoples and the federal government. Indian health is one such federal/provincial jurisdictional battleground, and the arguments in this case revolve around legal and political interpretations of the British North America Act (BNA) of 1867 (renamed The Constitution Act 1867).

The BNA stipulated that the federal government has a general responsibility for native peoples but also defined health care as a provincial jurisdiction. In B.C., responsibility for Indian health is divided up as follows: the provincial government administers a medical insurance plan in which Indians are registered, and the federal government reimburses the province for provincial medical services delivered to on-reserve registered Indians. The federal government also provides public health services such as prenatal care and other non-insured services to registered Indians on reserve.

In keeping with their basic political position regarding the non-existence of aboriginal title, and as a part of their more general goal of expanding provincial jurisdiction, the B.C. government seeks to remove the administration and delivery of *all* health care services for *all* provincial residents from federal jurisdiction. Minister of Health McClelland set out the provincial position in a detailed policy statement released in November of 1979:

> It is the belief of the province that the care of native Indians will inevitably fall under their jurisdiction....It is essential that the federal government recognizes the need to co-ordinate the health care of registered Indians within the context of the provincial system. Such action might aid the federal government in rationalizing the magnitude of its public service workforce, and it is essential that an acceptable funding formula be developed for this purpose....[4]

Obviously, this is not only an argument about political principles and federal/provincial divisions of power. It is also a very concrete competition for revenue, transfer payments, and jobs. This situation creates bureaucratic nightmares which in turn hamper to a certain extent the efficient delivery of services. There are constant disputes about whether the federal or provincial governments, or individuals themselves, are responsible for paying insurance premiums for non-status Indians, status Indians living off reserve, status and non-status recipients of social assistance support on and off reserve, employed status Indians on and off reserve, etc. etc. etc. In such a context, patients can easily come to be thought of as nameless bodies with various price tags attached to them. The provincial policy statement continued:

> Even though the federal government does provide primary services to a number of our white population in remote areas, the fact still remains that the province presently cares for a greater number of registered Indians than the federal government. In addition, the province cares for countless others of native origin who have left the reserves or have lost their registered status in some other way. The issue remains that inconsistent criteria, based on boundaries and a class system, determines the application of two systems of health care to one population group....
>
> All factors must be taken into account in the development of a basic level of rural health care, for all persons in remote areas, and this would necessarily take into account the special needs of native Indians....There is some agreement that many of the more apparent problems could be aided by giving natives more responsibility and accountability for their own care...but...this participation more rightly lies among all residents of a remote area...*If* the region is predominantly native, their majority representation affords them an excellent opportunity to influence the care they receive [emphasis mine]....[5]

The provincial government was prepared to recognize the "special needs" of Native peoples, but not their "special rights," and, in the final analysis they were prepared to discuss only those means of meeting Native needs which could be implemented within the context of a provincial bureaucracy. The provincial government would not, therefore, listen to charges that Indians, particularly, were not receiving proper care within a provincial institution, would not respond to the Nimpkish Band's and the Kwakiutl District Council's demand for a public inquiry into *Indian* health care, and would not entertain any suggestion that provincial agencies or institutions be structured so as to be directly accountable specifically to Native communities.

McClelland included a specific reference to the Alert Bay situation in his policy statement:

The recent events in Alert Bay highlight these issues and it is now apparent that the federal government's unco-ordinated efforts to deal with health care problems, independent of a provincial plan to rationalize the care of the entire population in that area, will only serve to degrade the assistance that the natives deserve.[6]

Gloria Cranmer Webster attempted to explain to Minister of Health McClelland that the provincial position simply did not reflect either historical or contemporary reality. She wrote:

Dear Sir:

If you did not know before, you must surely realize now that there is not one community in Alert Bay, there are two—one governed by the Village Council of Alert Bay and then the Indian community, the bulk of which resides on the Nimpkish Indian Reserve and a smaller number on the All-Bands Reserve....

Mr. McClelland replied:

My responsibility as a Provincial Minister of Health is to assume that we have in fact one community and one health care system for the Province of British Columbia....

II. A SELF-POLICING PROFESSION

Two days before the Ballam Inquiry panel released their final report, Margaret and Richard Smith had received the following letter from the B.C. College of Physicians and Surgeons, dated July 19, 1979:

At a recent meeting of the Complaints Committee of this College, your complaint in respect to the service provided to your daughter Renee, by Dr. Harold Pickup was carefully considered.

The Committee, after reviewing the material relevant to this matter, was of the opinion that Dr. Pickup made either

1. A serious error in diagnosis, or
2. If he made the correct diagnosis his management of the problem was inappropriate.

In view of the fact that Dr. Pickup has been investigated under Section 48(a) of the Medical Act to determine his competence, and was found to be competent, this case in the opinion of the Committee represents a regrettable and serious error in judgement and the opinion of the Committee will be conveyed to Dr. Pickup, and appropriate action will be taken by the College.

The procedure followed by the College had been to submit Dr. Pickup to an examination of his medical knowledge. In other words, they ascertained that he did know what the usual symptoms of appendicitis were and what the standard treatment procedure was. Reaction to the College's decision to allow Dr. Pickup to continue to practise medicine was swift, angry and well-publicized.

"It proves what we have been saying all along. Substandard care is O.K. for Indians. We are united and determined in our stand. This situation must end and Pickup must go," Band Manager Pearl Alfred told reporters.

Harry Rankin described the College's decision as the "most colossal whitewash job I've ever seen...how can an incompetent doctor with a drinking problem be found to be competent in the eyes of the College? Pickup has cornered the market up there so another doctor won't go into the area...There's no sane way the College could have reached the decision they did if they had heard witnesses...What the College's inquiry amounted to was they asked Pickup questions and decided on the basis of his answers that he was competent. That's a pure whitewash job as far as I'm concerned."

Vera Robinson said, "This means bodies can be buried without a signed death certificate, doctors can be drunk at the bedside of a patient, drugs can be prescribed that are not suitable, and nurses can go undisciplined. And what is even worse, it means Pickup is no worse than a lot of other B.C. doctors...and this really scares the pants off me."

Coroner McDonald told the press: "This decision isn't consistent with facts brought to light during the inquest. The least they [the College] could have done was to withhold their decision until reading a transcript of the inquest. They are insulting their own intelligence until they read the transcript...They should have done the jury and the coroner the dignity of studying all the evidence before handing down a decision...My jury spoke loud and clear...I attempted to bring everything out in the open and I believe I did."

Dr. June Mills, from her home in Saskatchewan, told the press, "A cover-up will do neither the college or Pickup any good. It's a black day indeed for the medical profession in B.C...The College can't fool people in this manner. The public is not so dumb."

Under the headline "Cloud of Poison," the *Vancouver Sun* of July 22nd editorialized as follows:

> The island's only doctor does not have the confidence of the Nimp-kish band council, the elected representatives of more than half the population of Cormorant Island...What would happen if a majority of the people in Vancouver demanded the removal of a doctor? He would be removed. What if more than half the population of the city of Vancouver demanded a public inquiry into something? Premier Bill Bennett and his cabinet would fall over each other in their rush to pass the order-in-council.

159

So what is so different about the situation at Alert Bay? Well, it is a remote little place up there off the north coast of Vancouver Island, in a constituency represented by the New Democratic Party. It has only 1800 souls compared with Vancouver's 410,000, and 1,200 of them happen to be Indian.

Dr. Pickup has served the community well in the past and he may well be as competent as the College committee has found him to be. But the fact remains that he was found negligent by a coroner's jury...and that questions have been raised publicly about his drinking habits.

The *Vancouver Province* devoted its editorial of July 26th to the issue:

The College of Physicians and Surgeons of B.C. appears to be suffering from siege mentality in its failure to explain satisfactorily its decision against suspending Alert Bay physician Dr. Jack Pickup...

The College is now before the bar of public opinion and its failure to issue more than the barest declaration about Dr. Pickup's competency raises a number of important questions... Its refusal to cite detailed reasons for its decision makes one wonder whether it's simply manning the barricades against political pressure...

Now may be just the right time for the provincial government to consider putting a lay representative on the College's council so that the public can have some assurance that its interest is being fully discharged...

And the *Comox District Free Press* featured a cartoon depicting a doctor painting over symbols of Alert Bay with white paint.

The Nimpkish Band received no further correspondence from the College, but Dr. J. A. Hutchison, Registrar, defended the College position in a letter to the editor of the *Vancouver Province* of August 2, 1979.

The College in this matter of Alert Bay and Dr. Pickup found itself faced with two issues. The first issue was the unfortunate death of the child Renee Smith. The complaints committee of the College, on which there is lay representation, and the executive committee reviewed this matter and found Dr. Pickup's management less than acceptable. Both the parents and Dr. Pickup have been so informed. In this regard the doctor stands in a position of double jeopardy—reprimanded by his peers and subject to civil action.

The other issue was the very basic issue of Dr. Pickup's general competence. In this matter the executive committee acted quickly and appropriately in the manner directed by the Medical Act which is their

160

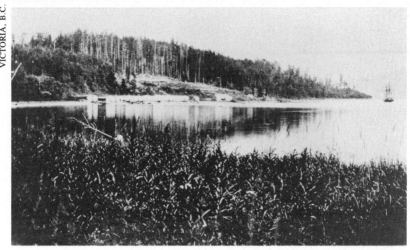

Alert Bay ('Yalis), c. 1865. This is the first available photograph of the village.

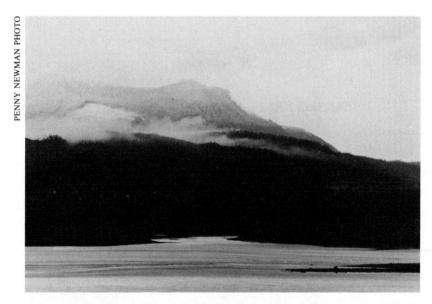

The mouth of the Nimpkish River (Gwa'ni) on northern Vancouver Island, directly across Johnstone Strait from Alert Bay, as it looks today. This is the original home of the Nimpkish (Namgis) Band.

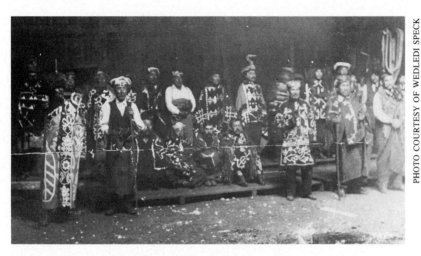

Kwakwaka'wakw chiefs at a potlatch, Alert Bay, c. 1900.

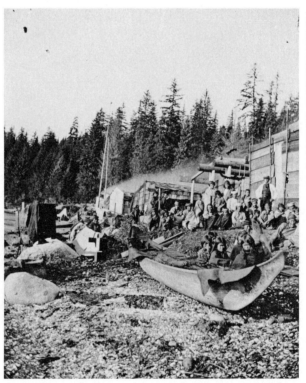

Kwakwaka'wakw gathered at Alert Bay ('Yalis), c. 1870.

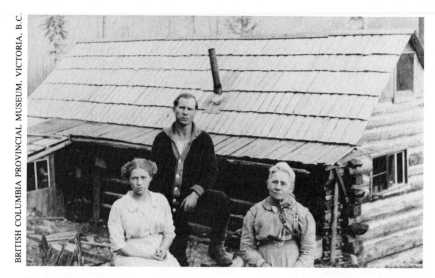

Typical loggers' cabin, Alert Bay, c. 1920.

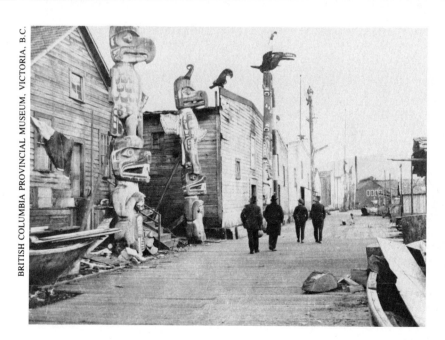

"Going down the road," Alert Bay ('Yalis), c. 1915.

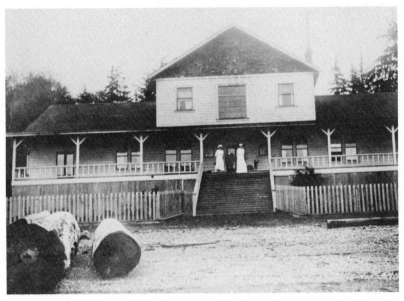

St. George's Hospital, Alert Bay, c. 1915. The hospital burned down in 1923.

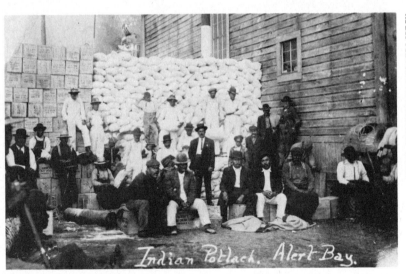

Potlatch at Alert Bay, c. 1920.

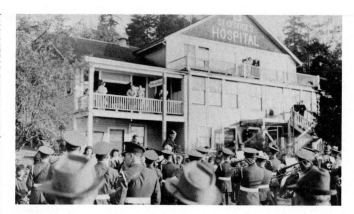

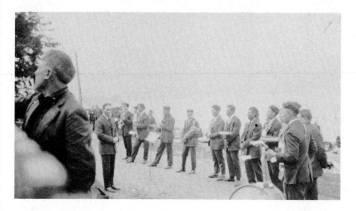

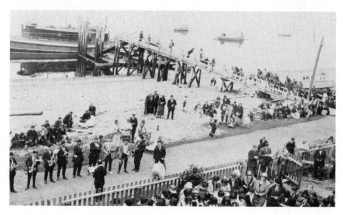

Official opening of the new St. George's Hospital, Alert Bay, 1925. Top: the new hospital. Centre: Indian Saxophone Band. Bottom: Indian Saxophone Band and students of the Alert Bay Indian Girls' Home.

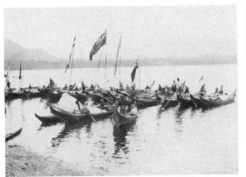

Kwakwaka'wakw from neighbouring villages arriving at Alert Bay to celebrate the coronation of King George VI, 1937.

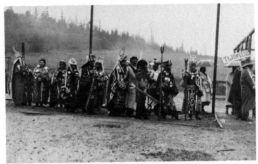

Members of Kwakwaka'wakw bands assembling for a parade to celebrate the coronation of King George VI, Alert Bay, 1937.

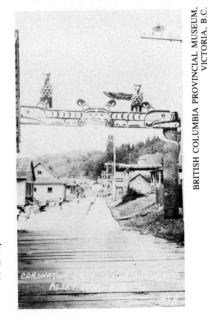

Coronation arch built in honour of King George VI, at the entrance to the village ('Yalis), Alert Bay, 1940.

166

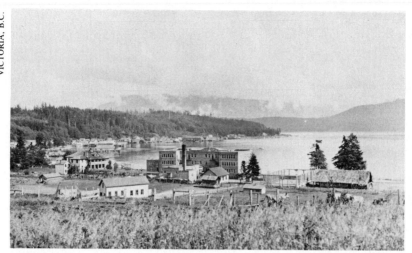

St. Michael's Residential School, staff tennis court, and farm, Alert Bay, c. 1940.

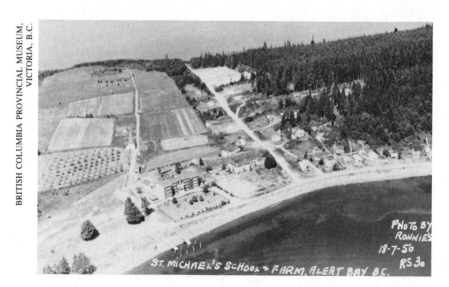

St. Michael's Residential School and farm worked by male students, Alert Bay, 1950.

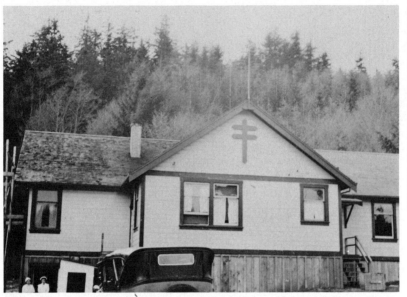

ARCHIVES—THE ANGLICAN PROVINCIAL SYNOD OF BRITISH COLUMBIA (ALAN GREENE COLLECTION)

Tuberculosis Preventorium at St. Michael's Residential School, Alert Bay, c. 1940. The "Pre" was built in the 1930s to quarantine students with TB, and it continued to be used for this purpose well into the 1950s.

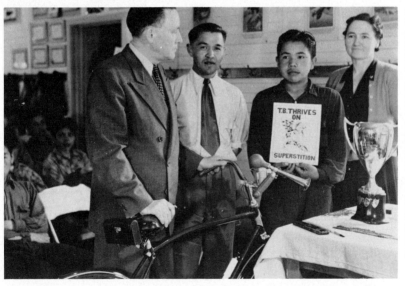

BRITISH COLUMBIA PROVINCIAL MUSEUM, VICTORIA, B.C.

Ernest Willie at the Alert Bay Indian Day School, being awarded a bicycle—first prize in a province-wide health education poster contest sponsored by the Department of Indian Affairs, c. 1955.

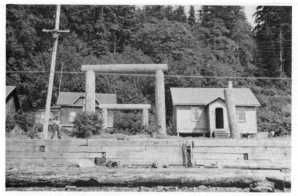

House posts from a traditional multi-family Big House remain standing alongside the nuclear family dwellings supplied by the Department of Indian Affairs. Alert Bay ('Ya̱lis), c. 1954.

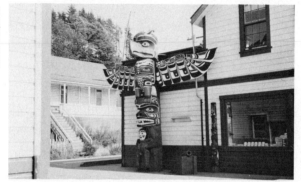

Totem poles outside B.C. Packers Ltd. store, Alert Bay, c. 1954.

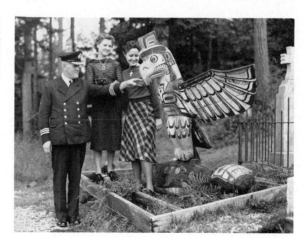

Visiting the Indian graveyard, Alert Bay, c. 1949.

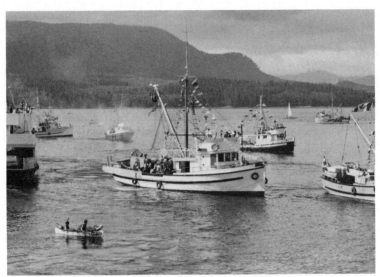

BRITISH COLUMBIA PROVINCIAL MUSEUM (ETHNOLOGY DIVISION), VICTORIA, B.C.

June Sports Boat Parade, Alert Bay, c. 1970.

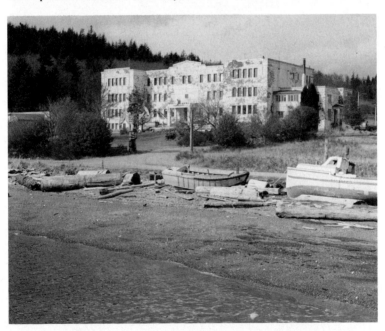

PHOTO BY DAN GILLIS

The Old St. Michael's Residential School, now converted into 'Namgis House, where the Nimpkish Band Administration offices, T'łisalagi'lakw School, and North Island College are located. The annex at the right, originally the principal's residence, served temporarily as a doctor's residence and Nimpkish Band Clinic during the 1979-80 crisis.

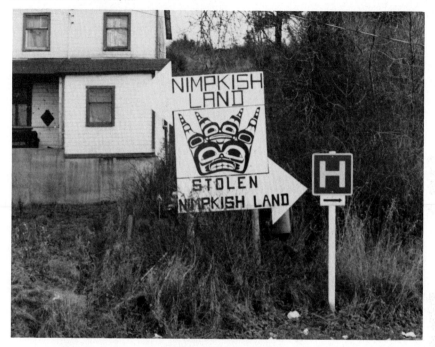

A sign of the times....Alert Bay, 1977.

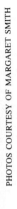

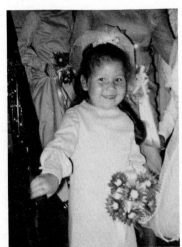

Renee Bernice Smith, flower girl. Alert Bay, 1973.

Renee, her cousins, and her maternal grandparents celebrating Christmas in Alert Bay, 1977. Renee is in the back row, second from left. Renee's grandparents, Arthur Dick, Sr. and Mrs. Nora Dick (now deceased), are seated holding some of Renee's younger cousins.

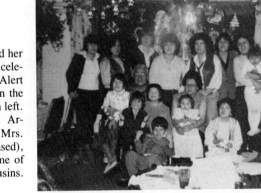

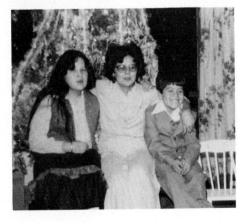

Renee, Margaret, and Richard Jr., Alert Bay, Christmas, 1977.

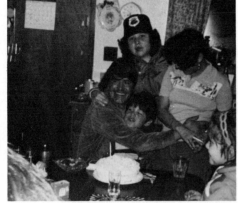

Renee and her family celebrating her father's birthday, Alert Bay, 1978. Clockwise from top: Renee, Margaret (her mother), a cousin, Richard Jr. (her brother), and Richard Sr. (her father).

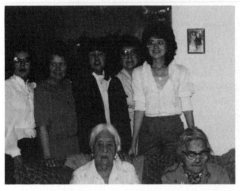

Renee's maternal aunts, her mother, and her great-grandmothers. Standing, from left: Margaret Smith, Vera Cranmer, Eva Cook, Ethel Scow, and Elizabeth Nelson. Seated, from left: Renee's maternal great-grandmothers, Mrs. Agnes Alfred and Mrs. M. Dick (now deceased).

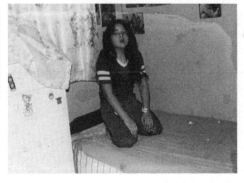

The last photograph taken of Renee Bernice Smith, Alert Bay, 1978.

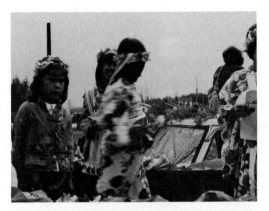

PHOTOS BY GEORGE SPECK, JR.

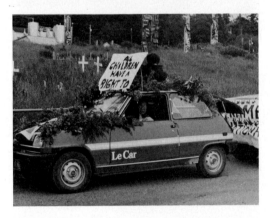

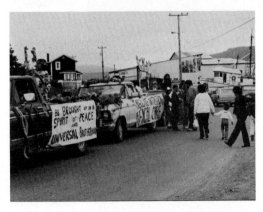

June Sports Parade, following the inquest into Renee's death, Alert Bay, June 1979. The parade's theme was the United Nations Declaration of the Rights of the Child, proclaimed by the U.N. to mark the International Year of the Child (1979).

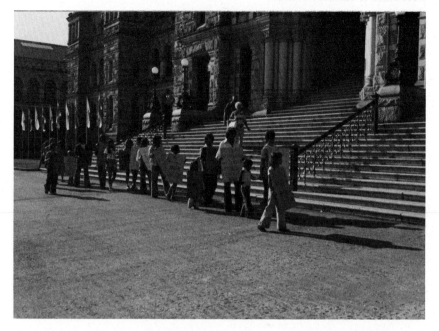

Demonstration at the Parliament Buildings, Victoria, B.C., to demand a public inquiry into health care in Alert Bay, and the suspension of Dr. Pickup's licence, July 1979.

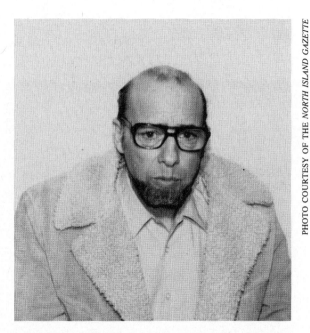

Roberto Enrique Trujillo (a.k.a. Dr. Robert Rifleman), Alert Bay, January 1980.

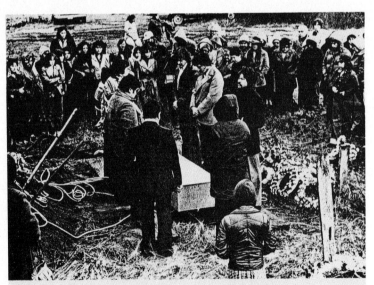

The funeral service for Roberto Trujillo, also known as Doctor Robert Rifleman, was well attended at the Nimpkish Band cemetery in Alert Bay last Friday afternoon. While posing as a physician, Trujillo gained the respect and admiration of Native Indians for his efforts in tackling chronic health problems. After he committed suicide in a Port Hardy jail, the band requested that Trujillo's body be returned to Alert Bay for burial.   Barry Bartlett Photo

Photograph of "Dr. Rifleman's" funeral at Alert Bay, February 1980, as it appeared in the *North Island Gazette*.

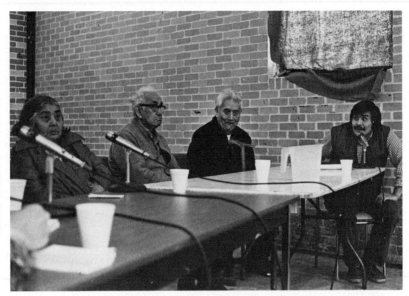

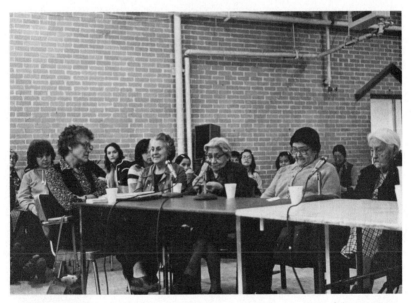

Kwakwa̱ka'wakw elders testifying about traditional medicines and healing practices at the Goldthorpe Inquiry, Alert Bay, March 1980. Top photo, from left: Mrs. Jane Willie, Mr. Jack Peters, Mr. Billy Sandy Willie, Mr. Robert Joseph. Bottom photo, from left (at table): Gloria Cranmer Webster, Mrs. Ethel Alfred, Mrs. Emma Beans, Mrs. Agnes Cranmer, and Mrs. Agnes Alfred.

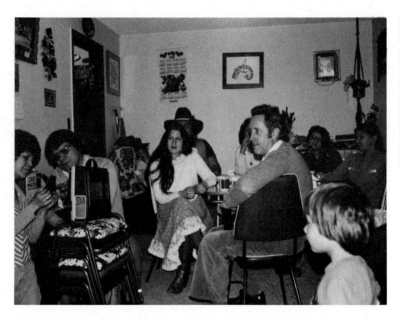

Dr. Goldthorpe, representatives of various native organizations, and members of Renee Smith's family preparing for inquiry hearings, Alert Bay, March 1980.

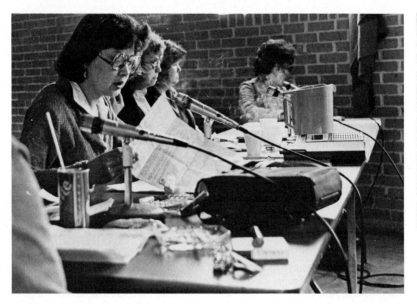

Renee's aunt, Elizabeth Nelson, testifying on behalf of her family at the Goldthorpe Inquiry, Alert Bay, March 1980.

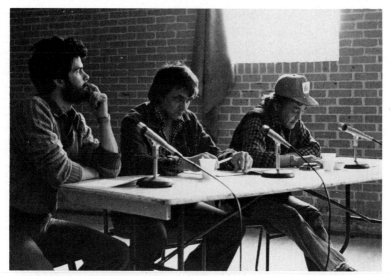

Kwakwa̱ka'wakw representatives testifying at the Goldthorpe Inquiry, Alert Bay, March 1980. From left: Wedledi Speck, Chief Bill Cranmer, Chief Roy Cranmer.

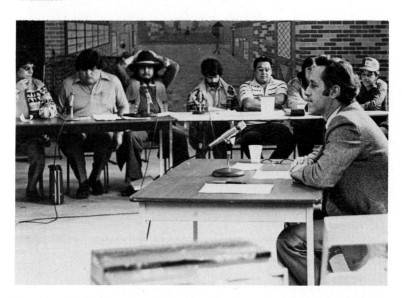

Representatives from various Native organizations and Kwakwa̱ka'wakw communities testifying at the Goldthorpe Inquiry, Alert Bay, March 1980. Seated, from left: Jim White, Bob Warren, Derek Wilson, Wedledi Speck, Basil Ambers, Ernest Willie, Chief Roy Cranmer. Foreground: Dr. Gary Goldthorpe.

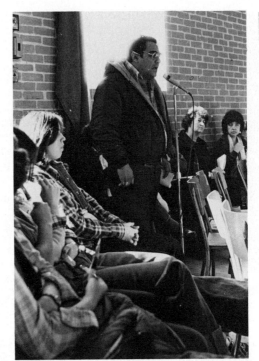

PHOTOS COURTESY OF THE *NORTH ISLAND GAZETTE*

Chief Basil Ambers testifying at the Goldthorpe Inquiry, Alert Bay, March 1980.

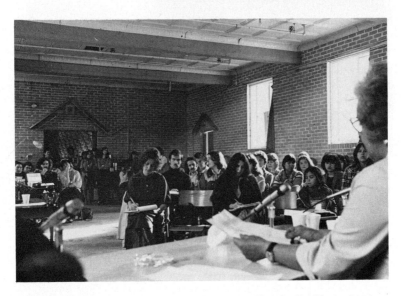

Community members, journalists, and visitors attending the Goldthorpe Inquiry, Alert Bay, March 1980.

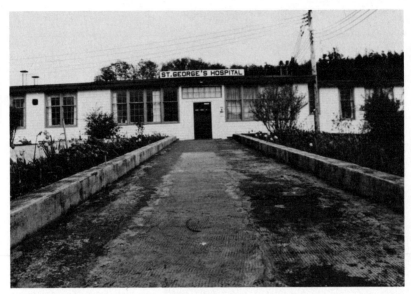

St. George's Hospital, Alert Bay, April 1987.

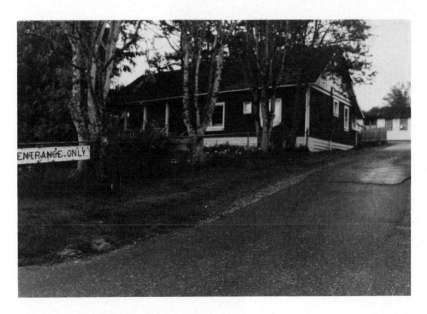

Dr. Pickup's residence, Alert Bay, April 1987.

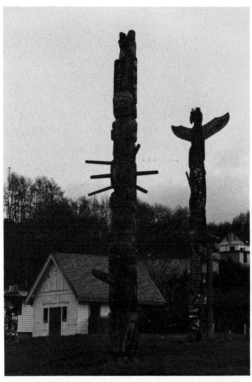

St. George's Hospital chapel viewed from the Indian graveyard, Alert Bay, April 1987.

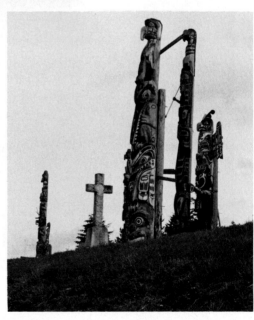

Indian graveyard, Alert Bay, April 1987.

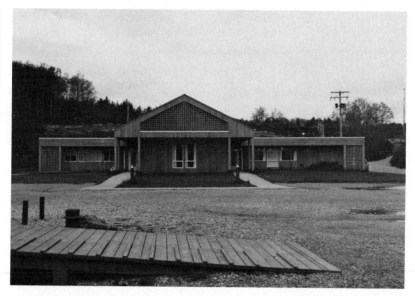

Nimpkish Health Centre, Alert Bay, April 1987. The centre was built in 1983 in response to the recommendations made by Dr. Goldthorpe following his inquiry.

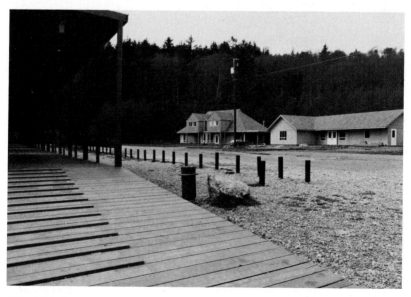

Nimpkish Alcohol Treatment Recovery Home (on left), Elders Centre (on right), Alert Bay, April 1987.

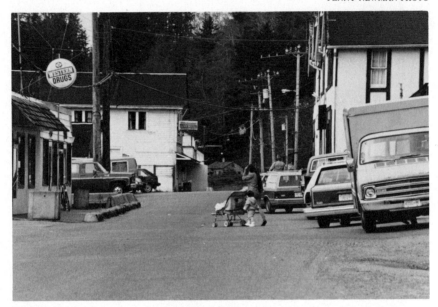

"Going down the road...." Alert Bay, April 1987.

authority. He was immediately ordered to present himself for examination before a carefully selected committee of three physicians who had available to them his entire file including the hospital records of Renee Smith.

This examination is an intensive examination extending over a period of three days commencing in the morning and continuing through late evening and covering both clinical and academic aspects. At the conclusion of its examination the committee reported unanimously that they were satisfied with his competence. Under such circumstances it did not appear to be indicated that his licence should be suspended.

In regard to other allegations, such as racial discrimination and alcoholism, I would add that no evidence has been adduced to support the charge of racial discrimination. Similarly, a letter on file from the hospital administrator in Alert Bay attests that neither he nor any of the staff have ever seen Dr. Pickup attending patients in an impaired state.

While to us it appeared that the fact that the complaints about Dr. Pickup and the medical establishment were emanating from a Native community played a major role in shaping the College of Physicians and Surgeons' response, the criticisms being levied against the College regarding their handling of the Alert Bay situation also exposed problems that permeate the whole structure and organization of medicine in British Columbia. Therefore, like the provincial government, the College of Physicians and Surgeons addressed itself to the challenges being made by the Indian community in Alert Bay within a framework shaped by its own interests in various political controversies raging within the medical profession itself, most notably: (a) doctors' rights to choose their places of practice; (b) the medical profession's accountability to patients in general terms of the self-policing nature of their professional organization; and (c) the concept of "patient responsibility."

A serious problem in the provision of consistent, quality medical care to British Columbia Indians is the fact that many live in isolated, rural locales, and finding doctors willing to establish permanent practices in such areas has been next to impossible. Although the Hospital Board chose to blame the Nimpkish Band Council for scaring potential second doctors away, finding permanent physicians had been a problem at St. George's since at least the 1940s. In 1975, the B.C. College of Physicians and Surgeons adopted a policy whereby, as a condition of registration, applicants would be directed to areas in the province needing doctors. Individual doctors challenged this policy in court and won. The provincial government then adopted a policy whereby B.C. Medical Insurance billing numbers would be withheld from new doctors establishing practices in areas already serviced by a sufficient number of doctors. This policy too was challenged in court, the doctors lost, and they are now appealing to the Supreme Court of Canada for a final resolution.

As a result of the primary resource extraction/company town nature of rural B.C.'s economic development, and the many small Native villages scattered around the province, B.C. doctors have always relied heavily on contract work for logging, fishing and railway companies as well as for the Department of Indian Affairs. Given fairly sophisticated means of transportation, doctors, particulary specialists, by flying in for short visits, are able to exploit this lucrative market without having to set up practice in rural communities. The recent, well-publicized controversy involving Dr. William Jory, former head of the B.C.M.A., is a case in point. Dr. Jory divided his time between practising medicine in B.C. and living in the countryside of his native England. He was charged, in 1985, with defrauding the medical insurance scheme by over-billing for eye examinations of Native children. His accounts showed, it was alleged, that had he actually performed all the examinations he was paid for, he would have spent an average of seventeen seconds on each examination.

In this case, the College of Physicians and Surgeons found Dr. Jory guilty of infamous and unprofessional conduct, suspended his right to practise medicine for one year, and fined him $30,000. The Supreme Court of B.C. eventually cleared Dr. Jory, saying that he had "performed the eye examinations honestly, if somewhat carelessly, and had no intention of defrauding the Medical Services Plan."[7] The College did not appeal the decision.

Meanwhile, medical care outside urban areas in B.C. remains a crisis situation for resident rural doctors and patients alike. In 1978 North Island Area physicians made submissions to B.C. Ministry of Health hearings into medical manpower shortages. All complained that the absence of a sufficient number of doctors in rural areas and poor facilities meant that as resident physicians they were were over-worked, under-paid and prevented from taking the necessary time out for rest and up-grading of their skills. Not only were permanent doctors unavailable, but finding doctors willing to provide vacation relief in outlying areas was also often impossible. These working conditions, an absence of "intellectual stimulus" and a general preference for urban life, they asserted, discouraged doctors from setting up practices in rural British Columbia despite the fact that "the income or earning potential might be far greater than in larger centres."[8] In April, 1986, a Dr. Kenyon of Fort Nelson relayed the following tale of woe in the pages of the *B.C. Medical Journal*:

> Since February 1985, we posted notices in every family practice unit in Canada, all major hospitals and telephoned each of the provincial monthly placement lists...We also were on the books of every professional placement corporation, made between 250 and 350 long distance telephone calls for a summer locum, with no acceptances. Many lower mainland physicians were available but declined to go beyond Hope...

Doctors resist the idea of being coerced to practise in rural areas, despite the obvious need, and at the same time there are, among their numbers, only a very few who feel any individual obligation or commitment in this regard. Well-meaning doctors will volunteer to go to the Third World, but not to rural British Columbia. Being forced to practise in rural areas is an issue that doctors apparently take very seriously. The Canadian Medical Association, in its "Declaration of Civil and Professional Rights of Physicians," lists the following as paramount:

(1) The right to practise where they wish.
(2) The right to decide their style of practice.
(3) The right to decide their method of remuneration.
(4) The right to be free of bureaucratic harassment.

While the delivery of medical care to rural areas involves a particular set of problems, ineffective complaint mechanisms permeate the entire organization of the B.C. medical profession and its relationship to patients throughout the province. When, in December 1978, the Kwakiutl District Council passed a resolution asking the College of Physicians and Surgeons to investigate Dr. Pickup, the College replied that they could not act on such a request but instead required patients to submit documentation of their specific complaints. This was made difficult by the fact that, according to the College's procedure for handling complaints, copies of such statements would be forwarded to Dr. Pickup. While he remained the only permanent physician in town, and the Medical Director of the hospital, many patients were understandably reluctant to do this. The Nimpkish Band staff, therefore, at first provided the College with summaries of the thirty-three letters, affidavits and signed transcripts which had been collected, along with copies of all the petitions which had circulated concerning Dr. Pickup. They explained to the College that most patients required some guarantee of protection from reprisals before they could be expected to come forward personally.

The College of Physicians and Surgeons said these documents did not constitute evidence. Furthermore, they added, they had received just as many, if not more, letters and petitions from Pickup supporters. The College said that what would consititute evidence was complaints from other doctors who had witnessed poor treatment. A list of doctors who had privately sympathized with local patients' dilemmas, doctors who had practised in Alert Bay and who were known to have witnessed events presented in some of the letters was submitted. The College did not respond.

Again, Dr. Jory's case illustrates the difficulties involved in pursuing any form of complaint regarding either the practices of individual physicians or the College itself. A number of British Columbia doctors objected to the way the Jory case was handled and circulated a petition calling for the resignation of the College's eleven-member council. The *Vancouver Sun* reported that "...Although the petition received a number of signatures, it was never turned in because the doctors were afraid of being singled out."[9] Apparently many doctors, like the general public, feel intimidated in voicing criticisms of the governing body of the B.C. medical profession, whether their complaints are about the nature of disciplinary action taken, or about the lack of disciplinary action.

From this evidence, it would seem that the delivery of medical care in B.C. is riddled with an absence of accountability at all levels. Patients seeking redress from the College are thwarted by the demand that they produce evidence which is often unattainable under normal circumstances. Doctors wishing to pursue complaints against other doctors or the College itself are too intimidated to even collectively submit petitions. While governments are prohibited by legislation from revoking the licences of doctors suspected of abusing public funds in the first instance, the College's disciplinary actions are subject to reversal by the courts.

Aside from ineffective complaint mechanisms and difficulties in locating doctors in rural areas, problems in the delivery of medical care to Native peoples also arise from the relatively new concept of "patients' duties to themselves" or "patient responsibility."

Patient responsibility is, on one level, simple common sense. If one takes care of oneself, one should, under normal circumstances, be healthier and require less professional medical attention. Increased personal responsibility for health has come, in recent years, to represent a rebellion against the monolithic authority of the medical profession and is seen by many as a way for people to wrest control over their lives away from professionals. However, some medical professionals have seized on the concept of patients' duties to themselves as a way of avoiding responsibility and as a legal defence against negligence charges. What is clearly two separate issues is blurred into one. While patients may decide to take better care of themselves, thereby gaining a little more power in this aspect of their lives, professionals often use patients' unhealthy lifestyles or living conditions as a scapegoat for problems in the health care system which originate within the professions themselves, or within society as a whole. Patient responsibility then *replaces* professional responsibility.

In the case of Native communities, it is particularly difficult to separate the interests of patients from those of professionals with regard to patient responsibility. Most Native communities suffer from chronic unemployment and social demoralization, which contribute to the development and perpetuation of unhealthy individual life-styles. Native leaders encourage individuals and the community as a whole to take greater responsibility both for personal health and for changing the conditions which maintain poor health. Conscientious medical professionals encourage greater patient responsibility as a means of changing the kind of dependency relationship which has developed over the years between the medical profession and Native patients. However, when medical professionals cease to consider themselves responsible for *health*, they too often also cease to hold themselves accountable for *health care*.

From a local perspective in Alert Bay, the immediate problem, and the obvious solution, seemed so simple and clear-cut. Yes, health within the community was quite poor and alcohol abuse was a major concern. People were trying in various ways to cope with these problems, recognizing that no short-term or miraculous solutions would likely be found. In the meantime, a doctor who was himself not similarly afflicted, and a hospital administration and staff that followed standard rules and procedures were needed. Apparently, however, the Native community was presenting the medical profession with a dilemma they could not, or would not, resolve.

III. THE COMMON FOUNDATION

> *British Columbia*
> *Thursday, January 22, 1885*
>   *Wacash, who has been affected with a vomiting of blood for some days past came last night and applied for medicine, but fearing that should he die his friends might demand payment as is the custom in the interior of the Columbia, I would give him nothing. Boston today pleaded hard in his behalf, but without effect. In the afternoon Wacash departed, in all likelihood offended.*
>   *It is a pity that the prejudices of the natives oblige one to withhold assistance, where it would probably be of service.*
>
> *—The Journals of William Fraser Tolmie: Physician and Fur Trader*,
> Mitchell Press, Vancouver, 1963, p. 301

The St. George's Hospital Board, the College of Physicians and Surgeons and the provincial government each had their own particular reasons for dealing as they did with the grievances being presented by the Native community in Alert Bay in 1979. Their responses were shaped in part by their overall interpretation of their responsibilities towards patients and the public in general, and, to some extent, they found themselves entangled in a complex web of legal and political relationships which they had, for the most part, inherited rather than created. But, when specifically dealing with Native peoples and communities, underlying this whole maze was a common starting point that defined the context in which all the responses were formulated: in the structure of Canadian society, aboriginal peoples occupy the position of a colonized minority.

189

This relationship has shaped the character of Indian/White interaction in British Columbia from the time Europeans first settled to the present day. It is this that allows Native history to be rewritten or ignored, Native lands and resources to be withheld from Native control, Native societies to be denied the right to govern themselves, and Native peoples to be deemed in need of external care and administration.

While colonization involves the exploitation of lands, resources and labour of indigenous populations by non-indigenous groups, accompanied by political and cultural subordination, crucial to the colonizing process is the development of an ideology which describes the character of the peoples and cultures undergoing colonization, justifies the domination of indigenous peoples by colonizing powers, and establishes standards which define appropriate treatment of the colonized.

The form of colonial ideology which remains prevalent in Canada not only reflects a desire for land, jobs and power, a denial of human rights, and a lack of respect for differences, but its most fundamental feature is that contained within it are value judgements based on ethnocentric comparisons between Euro-Canadian and Native cultures. A certain degree of respect for Native peoples and cultures has developed in recent years in some sectors of the non-Native population, however most Canadians still consider European-based cultures to be inherently superior, to represent the pinnacle of progress and human development, and to have evolved further towards individual and societal perfection than any others. Such comparative value judgements not only condemn Native ways of life, but in so doing they simultaneously glorify and idealize the dominant culture. These beliefs, implicitly and explicitly, unconsciously and consciously, serve to explain and legitimate Euro-Canadian domination of indigenous peoples.

Historically, European domination of British Columbia is not usually thought of by non-Natives as having been achieved by either brute force or the overpowering of indigenous populations by sheer numbers of settlers. Neither do the history books say that the settlement of the Canadian West was motivated by greed and legitimated by crude racism, as, for example the opening of the American West was. Rather, in the popular view, enlightened bearers of a superior civilization arrived, who, while having made some errors along the way, essentially had the best interests of the colonized at heart from the beginning. These "best interests" have consistently been defined as requiring the assimilation of Natives into mainstream Canadian society; in other words, denying the viability and integrity of indigenous societies.

Economically, this form of colonization has resulted in Native communities serving largely as consumers of goods and services, particularly those services such as education, administration and medical care that have been seen as crucial to assimilation. Such an economic relationship perpetuates an ideology that sees Indians as requiring cultural transformation or humanitarian aid to "raise" them to the level of the dominant culture, and that assumes that until they do so Indians are less able than are non-Indians to determine their own best interests, and to define and meet their own needs.

In this way, Native people themselves—and, more particularly, the needs generated by the effects upon them of European colonization—have become a form of "human resource," and meeting these needs an industry in itself. Until very recently, this industry, by definition and in fact, has provided employment almost exclusively for non-Indians.

The Native response to these developments has been to acknowledge both the desire for, and the need of, services such as medical care, but to demand the right to define and receive such services on their own terms—so they may be better able to survive as distinct peoples within Canadian society.

In the area of health and health care, from the basic definition of Indians as dependent and inferior peoples, flow explanations that most often conclude, subtly and not so subtly, that it is Native people themselves who are essentially to blame for the health problems they suffer from and for the difficulties that are encountered in alleviating these problems.

The relationship between the "White elite" and the Native community in Alert Bay is an illustration in microcosm of this more general pattern. For example, *History of Alert Bay and District* provides the following explanation for the causes of the upswing in the Kwakwaka'wakw population after 1930:

> The missionaries, besides bringing the Gospel to the Indians, taught them to have cleanliness and order in their lives. Their villages were not particularly sanitary....
>
> ...[C]ustoms among the Indians...seemed barbarous indeed to those gently nurtured, and thanks is due to the tireless Christian labourers of the Church Missions that the natives came gradually to give up practices such as the Hamatsa dance with its cannibalistic tendencies and the belief in the medicine man's power.
>
> When an Indian fell ill, he called in the services of the clan's medicine man. These men had a great hold on the Indian mainly through superstition. They were clever men who preyed on the weakness of the Indian intellect and quite ruthlessly held them in sway....Their grotesque actions produced no effect on the health of the patient other than a psychological one....It is possible also that the noise and confusion had a detrimental effect on the patient....
>
> The several things the missionaries contributed toward civilizing the Indian were cleanliness, better health, the beginnings of education, and the Word of God.[10]

Anthropologist Helen Codere, however, disagrees. On the basis of an extensive study she conducted of aboriginal health practices and beliefs, post-contact disease and mortality records, and developments in the delivery of health care to the Kwakwaka'wakw, Codere argues that:

> The attitude of the Kwakiutl...was fairly realistic. Although they feared death by sorcery they did not live in a world in which health was constantly menaced or restored by supernatural means. And when additional medicines and treatments were made available to them they were prepared to accept them and did accept them readily. There seems never to have been any reluctance to use vaccination against smallpox, and at no time do the Indian agents record any unwillingness in Kwakiutl territory to accept medicines or go to hospitals....
>
> Although the Kwakiutl were quite ready to accept anything offered to them in the form of medical care and were obviously in great need of health services, the record of the agencies indicates that very little was done for them in this respect....
>
> Sometime between 1924 and 1928 the decline of the Kwakiutl population was arrested. Since disease had been the principal cause of the population decline, the factors contributing to Kwakiutl health were what finally arrested and reversed the downward trend. Among these medical care was probably the most important. Kwakiutl ideas, health practices and sanitation were not of a nature to interfere seriously with the effectiveness of medical care made available to them and the turning point in the population trend was consequent on a real increase in per capita medical expenditures [by the Department of Indian Affairs].[11]

In the contemporary professional literature concerned with Indian health the emphasis remains almost entirely on "what is wrong with Indians," or "what is unique about Indians," physically, mentally, culturally and socially. The list of attributes of Indian patients made by the British Columbia Medical Association in their report on Indian health which figured so prominently in Dr. Pickup's and the St. George's staff's "defence" at Renee Smith's inquest, is repeated in article after article and in journal after journal in the health care field.

And, this theme reappears again in the political platforms and disputes regarding government policies put forward by provincial and federal governments. The provincial government exploits poor health, and over-generalized stereotypical images of Indian life, to support its demands for more money from the federal government to cover the costs of provincial health care services delivered to Indians:

> ...In this regard it is important to note some current statistics...Registered Indians have far higher rates of mortality than the total population....

Other problems centre around Native children. Native children can be admitted to hospital for treatment which relates to family conditions, including malnutrition, battery and the like. Once in hospital it is difficult to discharge these children because no one is available or competent to pick them up and continue their care....

Further hospital-related problems exist among older natives. A native is placed in hospital for treatment and then released, with the rationale that further institutionalization is not necessary, but home care would be necessary to maintain the health status. On many reserves, home care services are non-existent or inadequate, and the native is re-admitted to hospital quite quickly....[12]

The problem is not that these issues are not serious ones or that they are based on observations which are fabricated or untrue. Native people *do* experience poorer health than do non-Natives. Alcoholism, while not unique to Native communities, is a serious problem on many reserves. Statistics show that most Native people are poor and live in substandard housing with insufficient heat and sanitation. No one would deny that regular, excessive use of alcohol on the part of many adults, and sometimes entire family groups, exacerbates all of these problems. It is a fact that some Native people do not understand English very well, it not being their mother tongue. It is true that some Native patients frequently do not follow directions or medical advice, either because the advice is not well understood, or because of a generally disorganized life-style. Dependency upon medical care has worked its way into the daily life of some Native people and there are those who use hospitals like St. George's as rest homes and child care centres. Ironically, however, when Indians *avoid* seeking medical help, this too is interpreted as irresponsibility on their part. And when Indians deal with their ailments by means of traditional medicines, or by seeking help from Native healers, it is seen as evidence of backward superstition. Finally, of course, this list of characteristics and problems does not describe *all* Native patients, nor does it reflect features inherent to Native individuals or cultures. Where these problems do exist, they are the product of very tangible circumstances and experiences.

Rarely are the complaints made by Native people about the quality of the medical care they receive considered an aspect of their "health beliefs." Scant attention is paid to the attitudes of medical personnel towards Natives, and few mentions are made of Native patients' highly sensitive perception of these attitudes. Rarely is it considered that Native peoples' experiences of being treated like dirt, or being attended to by obvious incompetents such as inebriated physicians, could contribute to a pattern of avoiding medical personnel or not following directions. Neither is much attention paid in the literature to the lucrative venture that ministering to Indians in reality is. Indians' more frequent and longer use of hospital facilities is attributed *solely* to their own assumed inadequacies and not to the need for hospitals like St. George's to keep their patient-days statistics up in order to support its medical staff, their incomes and their social positions.

In recent years there have been sincere attempts on the part of many people in the health care field to encourage a positive and supportive approach to both the use of aboriginal medicines and treatments, and to cultural differences in health beliefs and practices. Explanations of the many social problems found within Indian communities now also tend to take into account historical and contemporary injustices that contribute to social demoralization. However, in the context of a society where difference is, still, essentially synonymous with inequality, it is too often the case that no matter how sincere the motivation may be to acknowledge cultural differences, the result, in practice, is yet another version of a "blame the victim" way of defining the problem. The assumption remains that questions concerning the delivery of medical care and questions about the professional in the health professional/patient encounter, are far less important. The microscope remains focussed in one direction only.

Good intentions notwithstanding, the problem ultimately comes down to a question of power. A people denied the right to govern themselves are also denied the power to define and explain their own problems, and, most importantly, to resolve them as they see fit. A positive appreciation of cultural differences will not be achieved as long as the context in which people from different cultures meet is an inherently unequal and unjust one where the powerful examine the less powerful more closely and more critically than they themselves are examined.

This contradiction becomes particularly clear in discussions of "whole health," or the way in which patients' entire social and physical environments affect their bio-medical health. Like the concept of patient responsibility, "whole health" can be interpreted and acted upon in different ways. Mainstream medical theory begins and ends its analysis with the individual: if more individuals take better care of their personal health, society as a whole will be healthier. In this way of conceptualizing the problem, individual life-styles are seen as the cause of poor health at the community level.

Opposing theories share concepts akin to those held traditionally by the Kwakwaka'wakw: if individual health depends largely upon the health of the society in which the patient lives, then the ills of that society require as much, or more, attention than do individual ailments. What is often forgotten or ignored by contemporary advocates of "whole health" is that in order for this to be effective, patients must live under conditions that allow them to also control their "whole life." In B.C. Native communities self-reliance in the area of health and medical care has been actively and explicitly repressed as part of an overall policy aimed at undermining self-sufficiency in all areas of life for over a century.

Now governments are beginning to respond to Native demands for greater autonomy by retreating, in a limited and piecemeal fashion, from some fields of Indian administration. Good health, self-sufficiency, and a revitalization of traditional healing practices are expected to blossom rapidly in the midst of ongoing poverty, unemployment, social stigmatization, and a denial of fundamental economic and political rights. At the stroke of a bureaucrat's pen, health problems which have developed over generations are expected to be resolved independently of other circumstances. The onus remains on the individual patient to change his or her personal life-style, and failure to do so is seen as evidence of personal inadequacy and as the primary reason for the existence of unhealthy communities. Native people are being given greater responsibility for health and health care, but still do not have the power to effect changes in the entrenched structures and relationships which ultimately determine the quality of their lives.

The demands being made by the Native community in Alert Bay in 1979 violated all the comfortably established boundaries for discussions about "Indian health." This particular "Indian health problem" had its roots in non-Indian society and in the relationship between Indians and Canadian society. In order for it to be resolved, Native people would require more control over their own communities *and* a relationship to the larger society that would allow them to have influence beyond the borders of their reserves.[13]

IV. WE (STILL) DEMAND A SOBER DOCTOR!

In Alert Bay, in July of 1979, all professional and provincial doors had been resolutely slammed, and locked. The band therefore turned all its efforts to lobbying the only official body that could not, at least officially, ignore them. Yet another statement was released to the press:

> The province has made it clear that they feel no responsibility for Indian health and since this is a federal jurisdiction we are demanding an immediate meeting with the Minister of Indian Affairs and the Minister of National Health and Welfare to discuss this situation which we consider an emergency.

Hearing that David Crombie, the newly-elected Conservative Minister of National Health and Welfare, was scheduled to meet with the provincial minister in Victoria, about twenty-five band members—mostly women and children since the men were out fishing—piled into cars, drove all night and arrived on the steps of the legislature in Victoria in time to confront both the federal and provincial health ministers. A delegation of old people happened to be performing at the Provincial Museum at the time and joined in the protest.

Mr. McClelland directed his driver to take him into the legislative buildings by a back door. Mr. Crombie, however, drove straight up to the crowd where

195

the "Little Red Tory from T.O." was confronted by dancing, drumming, button-blanketed old people, some wearing raven and thunderbird masks; and tired and dishevelled women and kids carrying hastily made-up signs which proclaimed: WE DEMAND A SOBER DOCTOR.

"I want to hear you," Crombie said and he agreed to come to Alert Bay in the Fall to do just that.

In September, 1979, provincial Minister of Health McClelland went to Alert Bay to hold a joint meeting with representatives from the Native and White communities. The Native spokespeople attended but were not permitted to read a prepared statement and left the meeting *en masse*. The White community's representatives rose to their feet, jeering and clapping as the Indians left the Church Hall.

Another attempt was made the following month, in October, to send a Native delegation to the Annual General Meeting of the St. George's Hospital Society to present the following resolution:

> (1) THAT the present constitution of St. George's Hospital Society be suspended, and that St. George's operate under the direction of the hospital administrator until such a time as a new constitution is drawn up that will reflect the social and political realities of Alert Bay and surrounding areas.
> (2) THAT there be a committee struck of the following community groups and organizations:
> Nimpkish Band Council
> Whe-La-La-U Area Council
> Representatives from Sointula
> Concerned Citizens Group
> Kwaquitl District Council
> Alert Bay Municipal Council
> AND THAT the committee undertake the drawing up of a new constitution for presentation to, and ratification by, the general membership of the society.
> (3) THAT the St. George's Hospital Society terminate the lease agreement for renting of space in hospital properties by Dr. H. J. Pickup immediately, and that they do not enter hereafter into any lease or agreement with any individual or group of individuals that would give them the exclusive use of facilities at St. George's Hospital for medical practice.

This time the Indians were ruled out of order by the newly-elected Chairman of the Board of Trustees, Coroner Deadman, whose wife was still the medical records librarian. The Native delegation walked out, again, and turned their attention to preparing for the upcoming meeting with Mr. Crombie.

The Minister of National Health and Welfare arrived during the second week of October, accompanied by a battery of reporters and photographers. Native people filled the gymnasium of the old residential school and told their stories and articulated their demands. Once again the press recorded the horror in detail.

George Speck, Jr. read a statement to Mr. Crombie:

> Mr. Minister, I have lived here all my life and although Dr. Pickup delivered me, I know that the charges against him and the administration that keeps him are true. I know that the 250 people who signed a petition asking for his resignation due to his treating people while intoxicated and his making racial slurs towards Indian people are not liars. I also know that people in your Department have, for many years, known about our problems here and have done nothing about it. Why? Is a doctor's reputation more important than our lives?
>
> You are the Minister of National Health and Welfare. You are responsible for the organization, delivery and quality of health care given to Native people.
>
> What are you going to do?

Mr. Crombie sat with furrowed brow and pained expression as he listened to the litany of horrors. He thanked each speaker in turn and expressed his deepest sympathy. One of the chiefs, however, left the Minister speechless when he asked:

> Is your system so fragile...is your power so insecure that you can't handle this one, tiny challenge us little group of people—and we're in pretty tough shape ourselves—is making?
>
> Look at us...We survived...We been just about wiped out...We been ruled by you guys for 100 years now and we're still here, still givin' you a hard time.
>
> Look at you...We say one of your old doctors is a drunk and we don't want him messin' us up anymore...We *prove* he's a drunk in *your* courts, and look at you. All hell breaks loose! You're all runnin' around in circles—investigatin' this, investigatin' that...
>
> I'll never figure you guys out!

V. GIVING WITH ONE HAND AND TAKING WITH THE OTHER: THE FEDS

Indeed, the federal government's response to Alert Bay's medical crisis would prove to be shaped by factors even more complex than those that guided either the B.C. College of Physicians and Surgeons or the provincial government. Since the Indian Act was first legislated in 1876, the federal government,

197

like the government of the province, has pursued various policies aimed at doing away with all aspects of Native peoples' unique legal and political status within Canada. Unlike the province of B.C., however, the federal government is bound by various treaties and legislation dating back to the Royal Proclamation of 1763 which it cannot simply ignore or reinterpret as it pleases. It is therefore compelled to seek some form of settlement with aboriginal peoples on issues relating to land claims and self-government. Of course, the kind of resolution to these problems which the federal government strives to achieve is one that is consistent with the ultimate goal of alienating Native peoples from their lands and resources and assimilating the Native population. They seek a settlement which will be both inexpensive and politically acceptable to the majority of non-Native Canadian voters.

The Native position is that aboriginal title and the right to self-government, must be recognized first and be the starting point for negotiating a new relationship with the Canadian state. Unless or until that happens, it is in their interests to defend their special relationship with the federal government.

Like the province, the federal government relies on the British North America Act to define its responsibilities concerning Indian health:

> The Federal Government has a *general* responsibility in respect of Indians as a result of Section 91 of the British North America Act which gives Canada legislative jurisdiction over Indians and lands reserved for Indians....The policy of the Federal Government has been and is that in accordance with its general responsibility in respect of Indians it should do what is necessary to ensure that Indians have access to adequate health services so they can achieve a standard of health comparable to that of other Canadians.[14]

The relationship between *legislated obligations*, and *discretionary policies*, is a controversial one in the field of Indian administration, since the federal government can, legally, divest itself of discretionary policies. Legislated obligations, however, being defined by law, are far more difficult to change. Once again, health care forms a major battleground. According to their interpretation, the federal government is not legislatively bound by the BNA or the Indian Act to provide special health services to Native people, but is only morally committed to bringing Indian health up to national standards.

To the federal government, with its long range commitment to withdrawing from Indian administration, "Indian health" is defined as a two-fold problem: First, since alcohol abuse is the immediate cause of the majority of Indian health problems and deaths, and is what most distinguishes Indian health and particularly mortality statistics from those describing the non-Indian population, alcohol abuse ironically constitutes a major obstacle preventing the federal government from declaring that Indian health is now "comparable to that of other Canadians." Hence, the Department of National Health and Welfare's Medical Services/Indian Health Division, as well as funding comprehensive public health services, allocates much of its resources to health promotion and education programs aimed at the prevention of alcohol abuse. The second part of the problem is that raising Indian health to an acceptable level must be done within budgetary constraints.

One of the consequences of the federal interpretation of its obligations in the area of Indian health is that eligibility criteria for recipients of federal services are also discretionary, as is the amount that the Treasury Board chooses to allocate to these services annually.

Medical Services issued guidelines to field staff, based on their 1975 policy, that set out eligibility criteria for people wishing to use their services:

GUIDELINES FOR OBTAINING MEDICAL SERVICES ASSISTANCE FOR INDIANS:

Medical Services receives funds to assist Indians living on reserve and those living the Indian way of life. In order to help those who move off the reserve to become established, assistance is continued for up to one year if necessary or until such time as the individual would be eligible for assistance from the municipality in which he lives.

Medical Services uses the term "Medically Indigent" to denote a person or family who is unable to pay a medical or dental bill because to do so would cause financial hardship to the individual or family. This means that a person may be able to pay a small bill but considered medically indigent if the bill for services were several hundred dollars. It also implies that a family with a moderate income and many dependents with considerable expenses may be medically indigent whereas a small healthy family with less income could be self-supporting. "Medically Indigent" differs from "socially indigent" in that it does not require that an individual or family be wholly dependent upon welfare for support.

Hospitalization is provided by the Province for all residents. A $1.00/day co-insurance charge is made. Medical Services will pay this for medically indigent registered Indians living on reserve.

British Columbia Medical Plan coverage is paid for by this Department for all medically indigent Indians on reserve. Those covered are also permitted to obtain drugs free from the druggist. Indians who are steadily employed are usually covered for B.C.M.P. at their employment. This coverage frequently does not include supply of drugs. If, perhaps because of the need for many expensive drugs, the person is medically indigent, a note authorizing supply of drugs as a charge against Medical Services can be issued.

Dental Work up to $100.00 for school children and socially indigent adults will be provided without prior approval. Other dental work

199

requires approval before the work is done.

Prescription Glasses: On reserve registered Indian preschoolers, school children and adults attending approved educational institutions may, with prior approval, be provided with standard frame spectacles at public expense. Subsidization of the cost of fancy frames for students is allowed up to the cost limit of standard frames.

["Fancy" frames are the kind a child *might* be convinced to wear in school. They look like everyone else's. "Standard" frames are the kind kids shove in their pockets the moment they leave home and then "lose" the first day they have them. They are the kind that bring jeers and sneers from classmates.]

There are constant misunderstandings and disputes over these payments as decisions about who should pay what are left up to field workers who often base their decisions on their own values and personal opinions about the "morality" of free medical care and which strategy has the best potential "retraining" benefits. Needless to say, between high health care staff turnover, paternalistic favoritism and changing directives from above, messages to Indians about how the whole scheme is supposed to work are confusing at best. The result, often, is that Indians do not receive the services they assume are their due, and are publicly humiliated about "wanting everything for nothing" and being a "drain on the Canadian taxpayer."

Again, in discussions of problems with the cost of health care delivery to Natives, we find no mention of the fact that "free" glasses, dentures, braces, prosthetics, transportation and lodgings are often provided through government contracts to specific private suppliers. Public attention, and indignation, focusses on the Native mother who stays in a "free" hotel room while her child is in a city hospital, and not on the designated hotel owner's coffers which fill up with Medical Services chits. Resentment is directed toward the Indian child receiving "free" glasses, but not at the optical firm with a government contract unloading out-dated frames at the taxpayer's expense.

In September of 1978, Monique Begin, Liberal Minister of National Health and Welfare, proposed significant cutbacks in health services to status Indians, which included providing benefits only to "indigent" (i.e. wholly dependent on social assistance) registered Indians living on reserve. In a press release, issued on December 21, 1978, the Department of National Health and Welfare reiterated its position *vis-à-vis* Indian health care:

There are no Federal statutes, including the Indian Act, which establish the right of Indians to free health services or to be provided with health services directly by the Federal Government.

...the aim of the present policy is to ensure that these funds, which come from the Canadian taxpayer, are made available to those treaty

Indian people most in need, rather than to provide to fully-employed treaty Indian people services which are not available to other employed Canadians.

The National Indian Brotherhood (N.I.B.), which represented, at the federal level, all registered—or status—Indians in Canada, was not consulted about these proposed cutbacks but instead found out about them in the usual way: a sympathetic bureaucrat in Saskatchewan leaked the information.

The National Indian Brotherhood objected to this new federal policy, and based their opposition on *their* interpretation of the BNA Act which, they argued, obliges the federal government to provide comprehensive health services to *all* Indians, everywhere, regardless of income. Indian Health services, according to the N.I.B. position, are a right and not a handout. Moreover, the N.I.B. charged, these cutbacks in health services were simply another example of the federal government covertly implementing their (officially withdrawn) assimilationist White Paper policy of 1969 which proposed transferring responsibility for Indians from the federal to the provincial government. If only "indigent on-reserve" Indians were to receive federal services, then all others would, in this area, be "considered as any other residents of the provinces." The N.I.B., of course, could not support any policy that moved in this direction.

Furthermore, the N.I.B. contested Medical Services' claim that the system was being abused and cited inflation, population growth, and bureaucratic inefficiency as the causes of increased expenditures in the health field. Pointing to the dreadful Indian health and mortality statistics as evidence, the N.I.B. charged that Medical Services was obviously not doing its job as Indian health was not significantly improving.

The National Indian Brotherhood launched its campaign for "Indian Control of Indian Health," the philosophy of which President Noel Starblanket described in the following speech:

> To be forced to live a life that is totally out of one's own control is a source of constant stress, and leads to weakness and demoralization of individuals and entire communities. We as Indian people have been forced into coerced dependence upon paternalistic and ever-shifting federal policies and this situation has contributed to a great extent to the manifestations of social ill health now seen among us, including alcohol and drug abuse, family breakdown, suicides, accidents and violent deaths. There is increasing evidence that the stress of dependence and uncertainty leads to physical sickness and disease as well.[15]

The N.I.B. position was based on two main tenets: first, that Indian health was extremely poor due to the stress of living within a colonial and dependent relationship to the rest of Canadian society; and, second, that non-Indians were incapable of delivering proper services to Indians.

The interim solution proposed by the N.I.B. to both these problems was for Native people to take control of the delivery of health care to their communities. They suggested that this process begin with a few selected demonstration projects which would serve as models for other Native communities.

In September of 1979, David Crombie announced that the cutbacks policy proposed by the former Liberal government would be officially rescinded and that a new strategy would be pursued to bring Indian health up to national standards. The new policy was to be based on the following three principles:

1. Recognition of the importance of socio-economic, cultural and spiritual development in attacking the underlying causes of ill health.

2. Reaffirmation of the traditional relationship between Indian people and the federal government.

3. Maintenance of an active role by the federal government and the encouragement of Indian participation in the Canadian health system.[16]

As a demonstration of good faith on the part of the government, Crombie appointed Mr. Justice Thomas Berger to conduct an inquiry aimed at determining effective methods of consultation which would insure Native input into their health care. "The federal government is committed to joining with Indian representatives in a fundamental review of issues involved in Indian health," Crombie announced to the press.

The Alert Bay situation was a dramatic example of problems involved in non-Natives delivering health care services to Natives. It was already well publicized, and a persistent thorn in the side of all the authorities concerned. Crombie agreed that an inquiry into health care, with a view to Native people taking over the delivery of these services within their own community, was necessary in Alert Bay, and could also serve as a showcase for the government's new policy. He promised to set the wheels in motion immediately. He would appoint a member of his staff to be the liaison between his office and the band. The Nimpkish Band's legal advisor, Michael Jackson, would, with the help of the provincial Union of British Columbia Indian Chiefs and the National Indian Brotherhood, and in consultation with the Band and District Councils, negotiate with the federal government for mutually acceptable terms of reference and the appointment of a commissioner.

Once a public inquiry was guaranteed, copies of all the letters, affidavits and transcripts documenting complaints against Dr. Pickup were sent to the College of Physicians and Surgeons.

A light was flickering at the end of the tunnel. Pearl Alfred told the press, "We are pleased to see that there is still some integrity at one level of government. We have some hope now."

NOTES:

[1]There are two hotels in Alert Bay and while they are located in the White End, they both have beer parlours and cocktail lounges which are patronized by Indians. Therefore, one cannot stay in a local hotel without coming into contact with the Indian population. Sometimes government bureaucrats and other visitors to the community choose to stay in the more "respectable" hotels of Port McNeill, which is, of course, a white town. Correctly or incorrectly, "staying in Port McNeill" while visiting Alert Bay is seen by many in the Indian community as an indication of a particular attitude towards Indians, i.e. either fear or disgust. When describing a particular visitor, it is often sufficient to say only that "he stayed in Port McNeill." No further comment is necessary.

[2]In the years since 1980 new administrative staff at St. George's Hospital have implemented and enforced many of the recommendations of the Ballam Inquiry board regarding the internal operations of the hospital and adherence to standard rules, regulations and procedures. St. George's obtained Canadian Hospital Association accreditation in 1984 and has maintained this accreditation to the present date. Dr. Pickup remains as Chief of Staff.

[3]"Status Indians" are those who are registered as Indians under the terms of the Indian Act. "Non-status Indians" are people of Native ancestry who are not registered as Indians under the Indian Act. While the Indian Act contains provisions for voluntarily surrendering status, the overwhelming majority of "non-status Indians" are women who married non-Natives, or non-status Indians, and who were, along with their children, thereby involuntarily deprived of Indian status. Among other things, loss of status meant that rights to live on reserve, vote in band elections, and receive federal services provided specifically for Indians, were also lost. The particular section of the Indian Act, Section 12(1)(b), which stipulated that Native women must lose their registered status upon such a marriage, conversely conferred Indian status upon non-Native women, such as myself, who married status Indian men. As a result of a prolonged battle by non-status Indians, this section of the Indian Act was found to discriminate on the basis of sex and was therefore in conflict with the new Canadian Constitution. Section 12(1)(b) was repealed in April of 1985, and Native communities are now in the process of re-formulating membership criteria.

Most of these "non-status" women and their children, of course, maintained close ties with their families of origin and their home communities. When possible, some remained residents on reserve, often living with relatives, or took up residence in adjoining non-Native communities, as has been the case in Alert Bay. However, *legally*, non-status Indians were not differentiated from other Canadian citizens and therefore, in the case of services such as health care, were considered non-Indian.

[4]Ministry of Health of British Columbia, "Statement on Indian Health Care in B.C." by Hon. Robert McClelland, *B.C. Medical Journal*, Vol. 21, No. 11, November, 1979, pp. 472-474.

[5]Ibid.

[6]Ibid.

[7]Mullens, Anne "MD watchdog drops case against Dr. Jory," *Vancouver Sun*, May 23, 1986.

[8]Brief presented to B.C. Ministry of Health, Public Hearings On Medical Manpower (Physician) Shortages, November 28, 1978, Campbell River, B.C. by F.K. Karter, Administrator, Port Hardy Hospital and Port Alice Hospital.

[9]Mullens, Anne, op. cit.

[10]*History of Alert Bay and District*, 1971, op. cit., pp. 20-24.

[11]Codere, Helen (1950) *Fighting With Property: A Study of Kwakiutl Potlatching and Warfare,* 1792-1930, Seattle: University of Washington Press, pp. 58-60.

[12]Statement on Indian Health Care presented by R. H. McClelland, Minister of Health for the Province of B.C., November, 1979.

[13]cf. Dyck, Noel (1986) "Negotiating the Indian 'Problem'," *Culture,* Vol. VI, No. 1, pp. 31-43.

[14]Government of Canada: Policy Statement concerning Indian Health Services, November, 1974.

[15]Castellano, Marlene Brant (1982) "Indian Participation in Health Policy Development: Implications for Adult Education, *Canadian Journal of Native Studies,* Vol. 11, No. 1, 1982, p. 122.

[16]Canada, Department of National Health and Welfare, *Statement on Indian Health Policy (Communique)* 19 September, 1979, quoted in Young, T. Kue (1984) "Indian Health Services in Canada: A Sociohistorical Perspective," *Social Science and Medicine,* Vol. 18, No. 3, pp. 257-264, Great Britain.

CHAPTER 8

When A Rock Falls On An Egg

There is an old saying
It is very wise
You can see the truth of it
Right before your eyes...

If a rock falls on an egg
Too bad, too bad for the egg
If an egg falls on a rock
Too bad for the egg.
—American Folk Song

Alert Bay, B.C.
October, 1979

It had now been nine months since Renee had died and the entire town—the Indian and the White communities—had been thrown into political and emotional turmoil. Over the course of the past year relations between the White End and the Village had become more strained than ever, and conflicting loyalties had pulled everyone in several different directions. The response of some people on the White End to the Ballam Inquiry and the report of Reverend Powell, i.e. that their findings and recommendations constituted a resolution of the issues raised at the inquest, and that *Indian* drinking was the main problem, had further demoralized those who had to deal most directly and intimately with Pickup's supporters.

There had never been complete unanimity on either side but despite all the rumour-mongering, threats and counter-threats, and the generalized hostility which had been engendered in the months preceding the inquest, both communities had, for the most part, been prepared to accept the solution offered by the inquest. Everyone believed that an objective, judicial forum from outside the community would review the facts and reach an impartial decision. It was now obvious that the jury's recommendations could not be enforced and that Dr. Pickup, rather than resigning, was in fact digging his heels in and refusing to budge. That nothing had really changed despite the jury's verdict and sympathetic public opinion was met by many with a "so what else is new?" apathy. Furthermore, Reverend Powell's entry onto the scene and the respect shown him by some of the old people made the struggle an even more difficult one for those who had to choose between offending and embarrassing their grannies, or continuing to defend what now seemed to be a hopeless cause.

Old people are influential within the Kwakwaka'wakw communities and no one enjoys displeasing them. When feuds or conflicts arise within families it is often "The Old Lady"[1] who will intervene and try to patch things up. "Old Ladies" are known to put their foot down when a dispute has gone on too long or gone too far, and when they order a "ceasefire," it is usually forthcoming. In Alert Bay, you are your family and to really fight against one's family or to stand outside it for any length of time is a painful proposition.

The Indian community, too, had pinned its hopes, regardless of diversity of opinion, on the outcome of the inquest, an outcome which had turned out to be a victory—of sorts. Nonetheless, the struggle had been a long and distressing one. The press had been intrusive, and for people accustomed to being invisible to the public but for their many problems and "deficiencies," the experience of watching some of the most intimate details of their community being described on the national news every night was discomforting to say the least.

In nine months, the combined forces of the College of Physicians and Surgeons, the federal and provincial Ministries of Health, the Band Council, the Hospital Board, the Municipal Council and an advertising campaign launched across Canada, the U.S.A., Australia and Great Britain had been unable to find another doctor willing to set up permanent practice in Alert Bay. Medical Services had sent a series of doctors on one-month locums, but many people in the Village began to grow tired of going to a different doctor every month; grew tired of trying to explain themselves, sometimes in halting English; and, since Dr. Pickup did not keep regular patient histories, grew tired of trying to recount their medical histories to other doctors. They grew tired of, or were unable to, travel to see other doctors. Many began filtering back, some sheepishly, some ingratiatingly and some defensively, to Dr. Pickup. They had good cause to wonder if the devil they knew wasn't better than the devil they didn't know.

There were few households and even fewer extended families within which there had been no conflict over the "Pickup business." By this time, many people were beginning to feel that it was all over now and best forgotten. These people longed for things to return to "normal," and took the position that if everyone stopped talking about the problem it would go away.

As in any political battle such as this one, while everyone shares in the experience, there is usually a small group of people at the heart of the struggle. In this case, this core consisted of Renee's mother's family, a few Band Councillors and some members of the Band staff, and some members of the Band Education Committee.

Renee's mother, Margaret, and Margaret's sisters, Eva Cook, Vera Cranmer, Ethel Scow and Elizabeth Nelson are members of two very large, close-knit, extended families, and hence closely related to many people in town, some of whom were Pickup supporters. The "Dick girls" were also active in the Village's cultural and recreational organizations. Margaret had continued to work in the kitchen of the hospital throughout all of this. She is a shy person, not given to fighting, and the strain on her at work was tremendous, not to mention the emotional stress of having her daughter's death continue to be a topic of gossip. Eva was an active member of various groups, like the Kwa'kwa'la Arts and Crafts Society, had a large family and her husband was a member of the Band Council. Vera Cranmer was a Band Councillor, President of the Native Sisterhood of B.C., a Vice-President of the Native Brotherhood, a nursery school teacher, and mother of three. Ethel had one daughter, worked full-time at the Indian Health office, and was also active in other community groups like the Native Sisterhood. Like Margaret, she had to face tension and antagonism daily. Elizabeth taught at the band's Nursery School, had one son, and was particularly active in community recreational organizations.

Within the Band staff, the most active people were the Band Manager, Pearl Alfred; the Assistant Band Manager, Wedledi Speck; and Gloria Cranmer Webster. The Band Councillors who were most involved were Bill Cranmer, Roy Cranmer, Vera Cranmer and Chris Cook. With the exception of Vera, these Councillors were all commercial fishermen with boats and tenuous livelihoods to worry about.

The Band Manager, Pearl Alfred, had held her position for over ten years. When she first took on the job, she, along with a bookkeeper and a secretary, worked out of a little house on the reserve which had been turned into a band office. Now she supervised the entire first floor of the old residential school and her staff included three office workers, an Assistant Band Manager, an accounting department complete with a computer, professional accountant and clerks. Furthermore, she co-ordinated all the programs and projects taken on by the band, and had a family of her own. By September of 1979, even Pearl was beginning to admit that she was getting worn out.

Gloria Cranmer Webster, a member of the Band administrative staff, was also busy supervising the initial stages of building a museum to house the potlatch artifacts which had been confiscated during the prosecutions in the 1920s, and which were now, after years of lobbying, being returned to their rightful owners.

Next were members of the Education Committee, a small group of ex-band office employees who were community activists and had been involved in the various developments and conflicts during the1970s and were now immersed in the setting up and running of an independent school. The members of this group who were most involved in the "Pickup business" were myself; my husband, George Speck; Kelly Speck; and Renee Taylor. I was working as an instructor in a vocational clerk-typist training program administered by North Island College, and had two children. George and Kelly were completing their first year of university courses by correspondence. Renee was in law school and spent much of her spare time rounding up bits and pieces for us in Vancouver.

Staff from the Kwakiutl District Council, Basil Ambers and Ernie Willie, co-ordinated activities between all the bands at the district level. Other people, notably other members of the Band staff and a few sympathetic non-Indians, contributed their help whenever they were asked to.

Vera Robinson, now Band Alcohol Counsellor, was involved throughout.

We were the people who had circulated the petitions, who had dealt with our own peoples' support and opposition, with the White End and with "outsiders" like doctors, lawyers, journalists, MLAs, MPs, cabinet ministers and professional and political organizations. It was we who had worked with the lawyers during the inquest, and who had written press releases, compiled information packages, drummed up support from potential allies, collected affidavits, interviewed people and prepared transcripts.

We were all—with the exception of Vera Robinson—members of families in the community and therefore subject to internal pressures. We all had to go down the road every day. Some of us on the band staff and on the Education Committee were used to being involved in political controversies and our immediate families and social circles were all on the same "side." To this extent we were somewhat insulated from the worst of the local pressures being exerted on people like Renee's immediate family, but were more exposed to the pressures from outside the local community.

When we had so cautiously circulated the original petitions, we had steeled ourselves for what we knew would be an intense, and inevitably bitter, local confrontation. We didn't think we were politically naive, but we had been confident that if we could expose to the proper authorities, and to the general public, what was really going on in our hospital, appropriate action would be taken and the crisis would soon be resolved. By the end of October we had spent nine months living at an emotional fever pitch where sixteen-hour days were not uncommon. We fought the authorities on behalf of the people, then turned around and tried to keep the people together behind us, and then turned around and made dinner. We were burned out. We were angry. We were bitter. Most of all, we were frustrated. As we ran, full bore, into one brick wall after another, our frustration began to turn inward. We began to turn our anger, and the bitterness of defeat that we were feeling, in on ourselves.

On the other side, some people, unable or unwilling for whatever reason to take up or to continue the fight, and embittered and defensive about their position, became increasingly personal and vicious in their criticisms of the people who had "started all the trouble." Renee's family, enmeshed as they were in the community, were very vulnerable, and these attacks were particularly painful for them.

And, there was the problem of public spokespeople. I had lived on the reserve for approximately seven years by this time, and had had a fair amount of political experience prior to coming to Alert Bay. Since I had been involved in the initial drafting of the petitions, I had been the first "band representative" to talk to the press, and I maintained this position throughout, although others, like Pearl, the Band Manager, increasingly played this role as time went on. Another public spokesperson was Vera Robinson.

Not only did the prominence, on the public front, of two non-Indians, supply ammunition to those who wanted to believe that "outsiders" had manufactured the entire conflict, but it made some Indians uncomfortable too. For one thing, it was constantly being thrown in their faces by Pickup supporters, and for another both Vera and I had reputations and histories of our own in the community.

As a "white wife," I was thought of by some as having "too big a mouth." My "yapping off" at band meetings, as well as my involvement in band politics, was sometimes resented and seen as inappropriate for a "stranger." For my part, I found myself in what seemed a contradictory situation. On the one hand, I had made Alert Bay my home, and it was my husband's and my children's home. I wished to participate in shaping the community. On the other hand, I am white, not from the community, and therefore always something of a stranger. It is a fine line which often only becomes visible after it has been crossed.

Vera seemed to thrive on being a crusader. Since her radio broadcast back in April, she and the hospital administration had been involved in relentless statistical warfare involving mortality rates and the length of time patients were hospitalized. She had also persisted in her attempts to have the Registered Nurses Association of B.C. blacklist St. George's, and by this point in time, the hospital board and the professional organizations were refusing to reply to any of her letters. As a result of her involvement, she had lost her job as an Indian Health

Nurse, and had been hired by the Nimpkish Band Council as an Alcohol Counsellor. She shouldered her new job with the same energy and vehemence, and her heavy-handed approach was beginning to elicit more than a little resentment from her employers, her co-workers and her clients.

Although as individuals Vera and I came from very different backgrounds, lived very different life-styles, and saw eye-to-eye on few issues other than the one we were both involved in at the time, to some people in the Village we were both white women and outsiders who were interfering in matters we had no right to be involved in.

Some people focussed their ire on the Band Council who, they felt, were not being assertive enough in the struggle they were now officially in charge of. Others were simultaneously criticizing the Council for causing trouble that wasn't doing anyone any good, and for neglecting their many other responsibilities and duties. In response to the criticisms being levied against them both internally and externally, the Band Council and staff decided to deliver the information package which had been sent to all the authorities to each household on the reserve. Their covering letter read as follows:

> We are concerned that some feel that our past actions do not have the full support of our Band Council. We would like to say that we have not changed our position which was made at the District Council Meeting in Campbell River in January 1979. And it was best stated by Renee's father, Richard Smith, when he said "We don't want what happened to Renee to ever happen to anyone else, Indian or White."
>
> As the elected leaders of our community we have a responsibility to all band members to do everything that is necessary to insure that another unnecessary death does not occur. The knowledge that we the Council and we the community could surely have prevented Renee's death if we had dealt with this problem sooner...is something that each of us must live with.
>
> As we struggle with the authorities over our request for an inquiry into the delivery of medical services, we hope that each one of you will read this brief history of events to date and realize that this issue is far more important than a lot of our day to day hassles with each other, and that our strength comes from a united stand. The band clinic is open daily and non-Indian people are welcome.

Embroiled as everyone was in both personal and political disputes, some of us started to avoid social contact with the town as a whole. It began to feel as though every chance encounter in a supermarket aisle was a slap on the face from one direction or the other. We shopped at odd hours, very infrequently went out to the bars on the weekends, and socialized only with each other. In calmer moments, we understood why people were returning to Dr. Pickup and why so many seemed to want to be done with the whole mess. However, the pressure of continuing to fight with authorities who increasingly voiced doubts about the truth of our allegations and the legitimacy of our representation, led to a situation wherein the choice of whether to go on fighting or not became an either/or moral issue and a political statement in our eyes: Those with courage and those who cared about Indian people went on fighting. Those without courage or commitment to their people gave up. This attitude served to further alienate us from the community at large.

When Mr. Crombie made the announcement that an inquiry would finally be held and people began talking about taking over health care, some of us were sceptical. The proposition that "decolonization," or self-respect, or pride, or political autonomy, could be achieved by taking over the administration of services that intimately affect everyday life had a tremendous appeal in Indian communities during the 1970s, and those of us on the Education Committee who were most involved in "the Pickup business" in 1979 had been actively committed to these political objectives for many years.

Therefore we agreed with the National Indian Brotherhood's analysis of the causes of poor health among Indians. We also supported, in principle, their solution, i.e. Indian control of Indian health. Doubts were emerging among us, however, about how much the self-administration projects we had been involved in up to that point were achieving their goals. In 1975, the National Indian Brotherhood, supported by provincial organizations like the Union of British Columbia Indian Chiefs, took a position in support of Indian control of Indian education. It had seemed like the perfect solution, and we had started an independent, community-controlled school on the reserve in Alert Bay.

But what happened was not quite what we had idealistically envisioned. The public school administration and some staff, finding themselves fighting for their own survival, mustered their forces and did everything they could to undermine the band's school. The District Supervisor for Education for the Department of Indian Affairs, the man in charge of funding, was philosophically opposed to separate education. He did not go out of his way to facilitate Indian control of Indian education. The Band school was constantly faced with shortages of funds and with last minute changes in program directives. Many parents were reluctant to gamble with something as important as their children's education and, at least initially, the school did not have the support in the community we had expected.

We were beginning to feel that self-administration was a trap, and we feared the long-awaited inquiry was in danger of producing another "program take-over" that would sound ideal, and look good on paper, but would turn out to be a nightmare when we in the community were left to implement it.

A meeting was held after Mr. Crombie left to discuss planning for the inquiry, during which the following debate took place between those of us in

211

the "Education Committee faction" and the rest of the people on the Band and District Councils, and their staff, who were most involved.

We held to our view that securing Dr. Pickup's resignation and exposing and holding accountable those who were directly responsible would constitute a meaningful, local victory.

They argued that the issue was larger than this and was clearly one of a lack of Indian control over the delivery of health care. A takeover by the band of health services which would serve as a model for other bands, and would constitute another step towards autonomous Indian government, would constitute a meaningful, local victory and would have the added advantage of really improving health.

We pointed out that we had tried to induce people to join the St. George's Hospital Society in order to vote in a new Board of Directors and had been unsuccessful in recruiting enough people to do this.

They said this was because Indians would not participate, for obvious reasons, in non-Indian institutions. This was further evidence of the need for separate institutions.

We said that taking over health care was just another way of dividing the community. It would be crippled by red tape and insufficient funding. People in the community would never have real control. The result would be that Indians would be left looking and feeling like failures again, a fact that they would be reminded about every time they went down the road.

They said that these things take time and that eventually these band projects would be successful and would be in place when land claims were settled and Indians had real control. In the meantime, people would gain necessary skills, strength, pride and independence from running their own services.

We said that unless or until Indians had real control over their communities, it was better to leave administration—and therefore the blame for inadequacies—with those who still held the real power anyway.

They said they couldn't understand how we, of all people, could be opposed to Indians taking control over their own lives.

We said we weren't opposed to Indian control of Indian health. We just didn't want another "designed to fail" program from the federal government. Most of all, we argued, Indian control of Indian health was a separate issue. We had started out wanting Dr. Pickup's resignation, and some control over the hospital. We should stick to those goals. Offering us a health centre now was an attempt to buy us off. We were being co-opted.

They said the demand that Dr. Pickup's licence be removed would not be dropped. The demands were being *expanded* to encompass the real heart of the matter: Indian control. They said the alternative to running our own health services was accepting things as they were and giving up.

We said the alternative was to continue fighting and to look for support from other groups and communities with similar problems.

They said all other options had already been exhausted and things were bad enough in the community. The alternative of perpetuating the conflict at the local level held little, if any, appeal, and wouldn't produce any practical, positive results, whereas our own clinic would. We were on a vendetta, they said, and had lost our perspective.

We surrendered but said we would not be donating our labour to the effort. No one objected to our withdrawal.

"We don't like confrontation," Pearl said. "What we're going through now is against our nature. But there's a limit to what we'll take. Indians have been literally helped to death. It's time we took control of our own health care, it's time *we* made the decisions about what we want and need."

NOTES:

[1]"Old Lady" is a respectful title in this context. The term should not be confused with the colloquial slang "old lady."

CHAPTER 9

Angela Richards

People they are different
Various paths they walk
Some are fragile like an egg
Some are hard like rock

If a rock falls on an egg
Too bad, too bad for the egg
If an egg falls on a rock
Too bad for the egg

Alert Bay, B.C.
December, 1979

Late on the afternoon of October 25, 1979, fifteen-year-old Angela Richards, a non-status Nimpkish Indian, showed up at Dr. Pickup's office. She vomited while at the office, and the nurse attending her testified later that she became concerned when she noticed particles in Angela's vomit. When the nurse questioned her, Angela confessed that she had taken a "handful of black and white pills" which she had found in the medicine cabinet at her friend's house. She told the nurse that she believed the pills belonged to her friend's mother, Mrs. Janet Douglas. The nurse checked Mrs. Douglas' file and found that tetracycline had recently been prescribed to her. She relayed this information to Dr. Pickup and showed him a sample of Angela's vomit. Dr. Pickup didn't order the vomit to be submitted to the hospital lab for testing so the nurse disposed of it.

When Dr. Pickup examined Angela she told him she had taken about 30 pills "last night," that she had not taken any other drugs, and that she had thrown up the first time that morning. Angela was admitted to St. George's Hospital with the diagnosis "O.D. Tetracycline."

She died, in hospital, thirty hours later.

An autopsy showed that Angela had died from an almost non-existent blood sugar level resulting from an overdose of tolbutamide. Tolbutamide is a drug used to lower blood sugar levels in diabetics and, while Angela also had tetracycline in her system when she died, it was the tolbutamide that had induced the "hypoglycemic encephalopathy" the autopsy cited as the immediate cause of death. Dr. Pickup had also prescribed tolbutamide to a Mr. Henry Paul, who was also a resident of the house where Angela told the doctor she had obtained the pills. Dr. Pickup testified later that since he didn't know that Mr. Paul was staying at Mrs. Douglas' home at the time, it had not occurred to him to check Mr. Paul's chart.

Dr. Pickup ordered three drugs to be administered to Angela when she was admitted to hospital: Dramamine for nausea and Demerol and Sparine for pain and discomfort. Since Angela had told him she had thrown up during the day, and since he had not noticed anything he thought was significant in her vomit, Dr. Pickup concluded that it was not necessary to pump her stomach. Urinalysis and hemoglobin tests were routinely conducted whenever a patient was admitted to St. George's, but since Dr. Pickup did not indicate that Angela's case was an emergency, these tests were postponed until the following day when they could be done by the hospital lab during regular working hours. (Although, as it turned out, the urinalysis never was completed.) Dr. Pickup checked on Angela before he went home for the day at around 5:30 p.m. Her guardian, a Native woman who was matron of the Receiving Home where Angela lived, was visiting her and Angela appeared to Dr. Pickup to be feeling much better than when he had seen her an hour before in his office.

Around 8:00 on the following morning, October 26th, one of the nurses called Dr. Pickup and asked him to come to the hospital immediately. Angela's condition had worsened during the night, presumably after the effects of the drugs administered when she was admitted to the hospital had worn off. The nurses had checked the *Compendium of Pharmaceuticals and Specialities* and had determined by themselves that her symptoms were not consistent with an overdose of tetracycline. At 8:00 a.m. she had begun to have convulsions. At 8:15 a.m., when Dr. Pickup arrived at the hospital, Angela's convulsions had ceased and her condition appeared stable. He said later that at that point he thought she may have had an "epileptic-type seizure" and he also considered possible head injury.

216

Dr. Pickup went home for breakfast and returned to the hospital at around 9:00 a.m. by which time Angela's convulsions had begun again. He agreed with the nurses that Angela was not exhibiting the symptoms of tetracycline overdose and that it was likely that she had taken some other drugs. He did not, however, alter his official diagnosis. The nurses told him Angela had had visitors the night before and although neither he nor the nurses knew any of them by name, Dr. Pickup concluded that her visitors had probably given Angela other drugs. One of Angela's aunts who worked in the hospital came to see her and Dr. Pickup asked her to go to the house where Angela said she had found the pills and see if there were any other empty vials. No one was home at Janet Douglas' and the doors were locked so Angela's aunt returned to the hospital and reported this to Dr. Pickup. Dr. Pickup told the nurses to give Angela a small dose of glucose and saline and went to his office.

Around 10:30 a.m. the doctor assigned to the Nimpkish Band Clinic by Medical Services/Indian Health joined Dr. Pickup for hospital rounds. When they got to Angela's room she was having convulsions again and she was experiencing spasms in her feet and hands. The Medical Services doctor agreed that these symptoms were not consistent with an overdose of tetracycline and suggested she be given an injection of calcium gluconate. Dr. Pickup agreed to do this, but did not request a formal consultation or second opinion on diagnosis. The Medical Services doctor did not intervene in Angela's care any further.

By 11:00 a.m. she was still spasmodic so Dr. Pickup ordered 10cc of paraldehyde—a drug used to subdue alcoholics undergoing delirium tremens (D.T.s). Angela's guardian came to see her again and Dr. Pickup asked her, as well, to try to find out about other drugs. The Matron of the Receiving Home left and spent most of the rest of the day questioning Angela's friends and relatives. At noon Dr. Pickup checked on Angela again and she appeared to be doing fine.

Around 3:00 p.m. Angela began slipping into a coma and having respiratory problems. Dr. Pickup ordered penicillin. More friends and relatives dropped in to see her but finding her dozing they left quietly. They didn't question the doctor or the hospital staff. By 5:00 p.m. Angela was still in a coma so Mrs. Pickup called the R.C.M.P. At 8:00 p.m. the R.C.M.P. brought Henry Paul's empty vial of tolbutamide to the nursing station in the hospital and reported that when they had questioned him about these pills Mr. Paul had told them that he had taken them all as he had been instructed to by Dr. Pickup. And since it was an old prescription that should have already been used, Dr. Pickup didn't think tolbutamide was the problem.[1]

At 9:25 p.m. Angela died.

Coroner Deadman said that, in his opinion, Angela's death was a "straight suicide." Since Deadman was also the Chairman of the Hospital Board, the

Regional Coroner decided that he was in a conflict of interest position and should not conduct the inquest. A new Chief Coroner for B.C., Hal Murphy, presided over the inquest which began in Alert Bay on December 13, 1979. The press arrived in droves.

Coroner Murphy began the inquest by addressing the jury which was made up of six people from the Port Hardy area: three Natives and three Whites. He explained to them that the Coroner's Act of B.C. had changed since Renee Smith's inquest and coroner's juries were no longer permitted to assign blame in their verdicts. Murphy warned the jury not to be influenced by previous inquests, gossip, or press reports, and cautioned them to "Be careful. Remember that thousands of people all the way to Toronto are watching you." He outlined the case for them and asked them to "Think about what this girl did to herself on the first evening when she took the pills....Then think about her subsequent treatment."

The Coroner's Councel, Sid Shook, told the jury there were two issues before them: what information the doctor was given about the girl's illness and whether or not Angela had attempted to commit suicide.

A debate then ensued as to whether or not the Nimpkish Band should be permitted standing at the inquest. Dr. Pickup's lawyer produced a letter from the Department of Indian Affairs which stated that Angela Richards was a non-status Indian who was not registered under the Nimpkish Band, and argued that therefore the band had no legitimate interest in the inquest. Michael Rhodes, acting for the band, produced a Nimpkish Band Council resolution which stated that the band did not recognize these D.I.A.N.D.-imposed classifications. The Coroner allowed the band's lawyer to participate.

The first witness to testify was Angela's guardian, the matron of the Receiving Home where Angela was living. She stated that Angela had gone out without her permission on the night of October 24th and had returned home around 9:00 a.m. on October 25th obviously under the influence of alcohol. The matron had put her to bed and Angela had gotten up around 11:00 a.m., had been staggering and had thrown up. The matron sent her back to bed and made a doctor's appointment for her. She said she had never heard Angela mention suicide.

Next, Dr. H. R. Patterson testified about the results of the autopsy he had conducted. He confirmed that an overdose of tolbutamide had been the cause of death and that he had also found traces of tetracycline, Demerol and Sparine in her blood but could not say whether or not these drugs had "helped her or hurt her." The results of a blood sugar test would have shown what Angela was suffering from and the administration of glucose over the first 24 hour period that she was hospitalized would have saved her. The dosage of glucose given by Dr. Pickup on October 26th was too little and too late.

The nurses had complained that Renee Smith's relatives kept bringing her pop and candy, which was against hospital regulations. The antidote for the drugs Angela had taken was sugar. Had she been fed pop and candy, she may have lived.

The inquest was told that Dr. Gordon Butler, National Health & Welfare Director of Medical Services for B.C., had written to the B.C. College of Physicians and Surgeons complaining that Dr. Pickup had not formally consulted with the Medical Services physician stationed at Alert Bay and had further criticized Dr. Pickup for not transferring Angela to a major hospital which would have been better equipped to handle a drug overdose. Coroner Murphy ruled out further discussion of this letter due to a technicality of law.

Dr. Pickup took the stand next. He said that he had assumed that the diagnosis of O.D. Tetracycline was correct at the time Angela was admitted and had further assumed that if her vomiting could be brought under control she would be fine. He had not ordered her stomach to be pumped because she had told him she had been vomiting during the day and he assumed her stomach was empty enough. He admitted that he realized at 8:30 a.m. the following morning that his initial diagnosis was incorrect and when asked what actions he took to correct it he replied that he asked her aunt and her guardian to try to find out what else she had taken, assuming a teen-aged visitor had brought her drugs the night before. Given his suspicions, why had he not ordered her stomach pumped that morning? He didn't think it necessary.

He agreed that in cases where drugs or poisons have been ingested, and the patient appears to have little in the way of stomach contents left but is still very ill, the common assumption is that the residue of the toxins will have entered the blood stream. Why had he not ordered more extensive blood tests? He hadn't thought it necessary, he replied. Besides, he commented wryly, given the array of drugs that are readily available in Alert Bay, only the most sophisticated laboratory in the province could have conducted thorough enough blood tests to check all the possibilities. He agreed, however, that the blood sugar test which was called for in this case was relatively simple and could have been conducted at St. George's. He didn't consider it, he said, because "in his mind" he had ruled out hypoglycemia on the basis of the history Angela had given him and the symptoms she displayed.

Dr. Pickup was asked why he had not transferred Angela to a larger centre when he realized that he didn't know what drugs she had taken. He replied that the first night she was hospitalized it didn't seem necessary. Early the following morning the fact that she was having convulsions would have made evacuation difficult. She would have had to have been restrained. By noon, after she was given the paraldehyde, she seemed to be getting better and therefore transferring-out appeared unnecessary. When she slipped into a coma around 3:00 p.m. she was too sick to move. By 5:00 p.m. it was starting to get dark.

Why had he not formally sought a second opinion? He thought the informal discussion he had had with the Medical Services doctor during rounds was sufficient. Why had he not checked with the poison control centre in Vancouver?

He said he had just as much information on hand as they did.

Asked what would have helped him to arrive at a correct diagnosis he replied that first of all it would have helped if Angela had not taken the pills to begin with. Second, it would have helped if she or her friends and relatives had told him what she had really taken. Third, it would have helped if she had displayed more obvious symptoms of hypoglycemia. Fourth, it would have helped if the empty vial of tolbutamide had turned up sooner. Finally, he admitted, it would have helped if he had conducted a blood sugar test.[2]

Angela had failed, as a patient, in her duty to herself.

On the third and final day of the inquest, Angela's family and members of the household where she had obtained the fatal pills testified. Under the headline DRUNKEN WITNESSES STAGGER CORONER, Bruce McLean, of the *Vancouver Province*, reported the day's proceedings as follows:

> Bobby Douglas was on the coroner's witness stand, insisting that he was sober on the morning Angela Richards, 15, took a fatal overdose of Tolbutamide pills.
>
> Henry Paul, another Alert Bay Indian, sat in the back of the courtroom interrupting Douglas' incoherent testimony.
>
> "They were my pills," Paul kept saying.
>
> The spectators, many of them Angela's relatives, looked at the floor, the ceiling, out the window, anywhere but at Douglas and Paul.
>
> "Escort that man (Paul) out of this courtroom," said the coroner, Hal Murphy.
>
> "He's our next witness," said Sid Shook, the coroner's counsel...
>
> Later Paul stood with the Bible in his hand taking the oath while he leaned on the coroner's desk.
>
> "It appears that he won't be of any help," said Shook.
>
> "I want him restrained," said Murphy. "Hold him for at least two hours... and make sure that he doesn't drink in the meantime."
>
> That was how Paul became the first man in four months to go into the Alert Bay lockup and why he never did get to testify during the three-day inquest...[Mr. Paul was never recalled by the coroner.]
>
> An outsider in town for the inquest and talking to Angela's relatives can't help wondering if the teetotallers in the Women's Christian Temperance Union are onto something.
>
> Booze is big business in Alert Bay, population 1,800, an island fishing community near the north end of Vancouver Island. The town has 10 kilometres of road, seven taxis, a liquor store and four bars.
>
> There is also a bootlegger operating out of a house bright with Christmas lights on the Nimpkish Indian reserve. The matronly proprietor gets $17 a bottle for the Schenley rye that sells for $7.15 in the liquor store.

The demon rum also looms large in Angela's background. Her father, Howard Richards, died on skid road in Vancouver two years ago. Her mother, Leane, also an alcoholic, died in Alert Bay last February....

Angela was living at the Alert Bay Receiving Home on October 24th when her closest friend, Elaine Joe, 15, dropped in about midnight.

They went for a walk, drank about 6 ounces of rye, smoked a little marijuana, then asked Doug Scott, 16, for a ride in his Datsun sports car.

He drove to the house with the Christmas lights and they bought what he said was a can of pop.

Aside from another brief stop at Elaine's place, he insisted, they drove all night without stopping. They spent 5 or 6 hours on the 10 kilometres of road until Scott wrapped the car around a telephone pole at 6:00 a.m. the next morning.

Angela, with a minor head bruise from the collision, walked with Elaine to Elaine's home on the reserve. Scott went elsewhere.

'Angela went into the bathroom,' Elaine told the jury. 'Then she came out and lay down on my bed and said 'good-night, see you, good-bye.'

Angela died the following night, after 30 hours at St. George's Hospital...

Coroner Murphy spoke to his jury before they left to deliberate on their verdict. "I strongly suggest to you that in light of what he knew at the time, Dr. Pickup's diagnosis and treatment were appropriate," he told them. "I would add that doctors are not supermen and we cannot condemn them for being less than perfect but only insist that they be reasonable and professional. In his treatment of Angela Richards that is exactly what Dr. Pickup was."

The coroner continued, "There is the background of a parentless child who lived in at least four homes in the last year. Even though she had relatives nearby, she became a ward of the government....I believe that you have to find that in the light of all the circumstances the medical treatment was appropriate."

After three and a half hours the jury reached their verdict. Death they said, was by misadventure, indicating they believed Angela intended only to make herself sick to get sympathy and attention. Suicide was also a possibility. They found Dr. Pickup's medical treatment to have been appropriate, "in light of the circumstances." The jury went on to list their recommendations:

(1) The St. George's Hospital Board insure that in suspected drug ingestion cases strict procedures are implemented to obtain full

information on the agent ingested.

(2) Renewed efforts be made by both the Indian Band and the medical staff of St. George's Hospital to bridge the communications gap and lessen the hostility that exists between them.

(3) An information and educational program be undertaken through schools and public health units on the misuse of prescription and other drugs.

(4) A crisis line operated by Natives be set up to serve the Native population.

To Dr. Pickup's supporters it seemed that order had at last been restored to the universe. Everyone was back in their proper place.

Somehow, the tables had turned again. Somehow, Angela's short and unhappy life and the problems her family had experienced, cast doubt on the public credibility the band had so painfully built up since Renee's death. Somehow, Henry and Bobby staggering around the inquest appeared to be more relevant to the coroner and to the press than the medical treatment, or apparent lack of it, that Angela had received. Somehow, everyone sensed that if this side of the Indian community's life was exposed, even the public sympathy that we had managed to hold on to since Renee's inquest, and upon which we relied, would be lost.

While contemporary Canadians pride themselves on being a charitable people and regard the simplistic snobbery and racism expressed by nineteenth-century pioneers and philanthropists with dismay, the poor in Canadian society continue to be placed in one of two moral categories: the deserving and the undeserving, and dealt with accordingly.

The deserving poor are those who, despite following all the rules and exhibiting all the proper qualities—to an appropriate degree and displayed in an appropriate fashion—of frugality, industriousness and temperance, still find themselves dependent upon the state, or, in the past, upon private philanthropy, for subsistence. They don't deserve to be poor and therefore they do deserve aid.

The undeserving poor are those who do not follow all the rules and do not exhibit all the proper qualities—or do not hold them to an appropriate degree or do not display them in an appropriate fashion. They deserve to be poor and therefore do not deserve aid. These categories of people are defined in our language according to their qualification for aid and not according to their material status which is undifferentiated: poor. Therefore aid may be made available to those who are deemed to deserve it, but may also be withheld or withdrawn from those who are not. Canadians may then continue to consider themselves a moral people, while at the same time preserving the belief that success in this society is ultimately determined by an individual's personal adequacy or inadequacy.

Since most Native people are also poor they are doubly stigmatized: as Indians and as poor people. However, in the Renee Smith case the Canadian public had been confronted with somewhat of an anomaly: the death of an innocent child who was a member of a large, recognizably loving, hardworking, and successful family who enjoyed the respect of their own community and sectors of the non-Indian community. That they should be treated the way they were was unacceptable, and somewhat threatening, because they had done nothing to *deserve* the treatment they had received. Their strength, respectability and magnanimity contrasted sharply with the doctor's drinking and the hospital staff's disregard for procedural rules and regulations.

But Angela was different. In her case the public saw another side of the Native reality. Hers was an Indian story that fit the mold. Her parents were alcoholics. She moved around. She was a ward of the government. She stayed out all night. She drank rye. She smoked marijuana. She did what millions of other Canadian teen-agers do, but she did it on an Indian reserve. Angela had not, as much as Renee had, *deserved* proper treatment. Hence the coroner's references, in his summation to the jury, to her family's history and to her being a ward of the government, living in a receiving home. These aspects of her life may have contributed to Angela swallowing the pills to begin with, but it is a curious logic that proposes that a teen-aged girl who overdosed and then went to the hospital for the obvious reason that she did not want to die, and lay in a hospital bed for thirty hours, was still, somehow, responsible for her own death.

Within the Indian community too such a double standard finds a certain degree of acceptance in some sectors. Aboriginal society was stratified and these divisions continue to influence an individual's or a family's status. And, there are some contemporary fishermen and their wives who will tell you, with pride, that *they* have never been on welfare and that many of those who are, are lazy or alcoholic or both, and therefore deserve what they get. Then too, for those Indians striving for upward mobility, the struggle required to change negative images of Indians in the public eye, of necessity, involves differentiating themselves from less fortunate members of the group—"we're not *all* like that." This often leads to a sense of embarrassment and annoyance when other Indians behave in ways that reinforce common negative stereotypes.

The Nimpkish Band Council had demanded and won legal standing at Angela's inquest. Their lawyer, Michael Rhodes, did his best, but few local people attended. Everyone in the community grieved Angela's death, but there was no parade and no potlatch for Angela.

While all these factors played a role in the community's response to Angela's death, the major source of the defeatism which hung over the Village now came from the fact that the battle, and the victory—such as it was—had been fought and won using "moral" weapons.

Indians are a minority people. Officially, they constitute only 5 per cent of the Canadian population. They are relatively powerless, and the political choices available to them for defending their interests are limited. Indians cannot use withdrawal of labour as a bargaining tool; most are unemployed. They are not numerous enough, and they are scattered across too wide a geographical territory, to defend themselves by force of numbers. Given their unique historical and legal relationship to the Canadian state, and the relative, formal independence of the courts, legal battles offer some possibility of success. However, fundamentally, Indians must fight their political battles in institutions and forums dominated by Canadian middle-class morality, and must invariably rely heavily on public sympathy for support to even get a hearing. During times of relative prosperity, like the 1960s, political messages based on the injustice of Indian poverty within the midst of an affluent society found a supportive audience. Now, during the recession-ridden 1980s, such a message falls on deaf ears; people are concerned with their own economic security.

Since World War II Indians have slowly and unevenly moved, at least officially, from being "undeserving" to being "deserving." Previously their poverty was crudely explained by their presumed biological or cultural inferiority and the option available to the "deserving" among them was to cease being Indian. In recent decades, as these explanations gradually lost credibility and acceptability to varying degrees, Indian poverty, failure to assimilate, and "social problems" have come to be seen as arising at least in part from the unjust treatment they received—historically—but which was now being rectified. "The condition of Canada's Indians," understood as having been caused not by the inadequacies of Indians themselves but by racial injustice, has been a glaring contradiction within the pluralist democracy Canadians believe they live in. This "morality," this guilt and embarrassment, this evidence that something is wrong with the system, has been an important part of the political capital that Indians have been able to use to assert their rights in recent years. This strategy has been referred to as "the politics of embarrassment."[3]

> Tiny encapsulated remnant populations...have access to few material sanctions...[Their] major political asset...becomes the ideology of the colonizers and the colonizeds' own skill in manipulating the symbols of their dominators; the threat of material sanctions is replaced by the threat of political embarrassment, through pointing up discrepancies between professed ideology and actual behaviour...The resulting power is tenuous and fluctuating...and it depends on the receptivity of some audience—elements in the wider society willing to listen to the message being sent by the dominated group.[4]

Angela's death and the publicity surrounding her inquest were felt as a defeat, particularly by those of us who were most involved in both the Education Committee and the "Pickup business." Angela was a student in the band's independent school, and she had slipped away right under our noses. What good was it having our own school? We had failed to insure that what happened to Renee "never happened to anyone else again." What good was it fighting for better medical care? Finally, we felt we had lost our last hope: public sympathy and moral outrage. Our sensitivity to this political strategy, fine-tuned by a decade of fighting on the front lines of it, now threatened to consume us.

Embarrassed, ashamed, demoralized and war weary, the community retreated into itself to lick its wounds. Some were angry at the press, some at those who had brought them in in the first place. Most people just didn't want to think about it or talk about it any more. The Conservative government had toppled, leaving even the public inquiry into medical care that David Crombie had promised—the last fragile straw many were clinging to—in doubt. It had been a year since Renee had died and really, what had happened? What had changed? Maybe Indians never could win. Maybe kicking up a stink did just make things worse. It was Christmas after all and it would be nice if there were no fights among the family over old Pickup.

No one in this Native community exists as an isolated individual. Everyone is someone else's mother, father, brother, sister, son, daughter, husband, wife, aunt, uncle, cousin, grandmother, grandfather, in-law. Experiences, no matter how personal in nature, are a property of the collectivity. No one remains untouched by either good times or bad ones. It was these bonds that had mobilized even those who were reluctant and afraid to sign the original petitions. These were the ties that had united people in the face of the "outside" even when internal disputes raged. Now, it was a sense of collective defeat that made everyone want to run and hide.

NOTES:

While the story told in this chapter was reported in detail in the daily press and was entered into the public record at *The Goldthorpe Inquiry*, neither "Angela" nor her family voluntarily chose this publicity and, in consideration of their feelings, I have referred to them by means of pseudonyms throughout the chapter. The names "Angela Richards," "Henry Paul," "Bobby Douglas," "Janet Douglas," "Howard Richards," "Leane Richards," "Elaine Joe" and "Doug Scott" are pseudonyms.

[1]This account is based primarily on a tape recording of Dr. Pickup's testimony at "Inquest into the death of 'Angela Richards'" held at Alert Bay Coroner's Court, December 1979.

[2]Ibid.

[3]Paine, Robert (1977) (ed) *The White Arctic: anthropological essays on tutelage and ethnicity*, St. John's Newfoundland: Institute of Social and Economic Research, Memorial University.

[4]Gartrell, B. (1986) "Colonialism and the Fourth World," *Culture*, Vol. VI, No. 1, pp. 3-18.

CHAPTER 10

At Last...A Sober Doctor

The rock it is not broken
And is most insolent
Must be nice to be a rock
For it is evident
That...

If a rock falls on an egg
Too bad, too bad for the egg
If an egg falls on a rock
Too bad for the egg.

Alert Bay, B.C.
February, 1980

Some time in September of 1979 a lanky, soft-spoken, middle-aged man had appeared on the doorstep of the Nimpkish Band office and introduced himself to the Assistant Band Manager, Wedledi Speck, as Dr. Robert Rifleman, of Wisconsin, U.S.A. He and his new wife, Claudia, were on their honeymoon, and, having heard about all the troubles in Alert Bay, had dropped in to take a look. Dr. Rifleman told Wedledi that he had served in the American army medical corps in Vietnam and now wanted to settle down in a quiet little place as far away from the military as he could get. Wedledi liked him right away. He took him on a tour of the island and told him all about Alert Bay, Dr. Pickup, and everything that had happened. The next day Dr. Rifleman announced that he had fallen in love with the community and would look into the possibility of immigrating.

The College of Physicians and Surgeons reviewed Dr. Rifleman's credentials and issued him a B.C. medical licence in record time. The immigration department, with lightning speed, granted him landed immigrant status. Scarcely six weeks later, in mid-November, Dr. Rifleman and his wife moved into a little house in the municipality. He introduced himself to the Band Council and made arrangements to work part-time out of the band clinic on the reserve. Then he moved into the spare office for "second doctors" in Dr. Pickup's clinic, secured hospital privileges from the Board of Trustees of St. George's, hung his diplomas and a photograph of the destroyer he had served on in 'Nam' up on his office wall, placed a framed picture of his wife on his desk, and opened for business.

Only another face in what had been a long series of new doctors, Dr. Rifleman found that patients were slow to come at first. He did, however, quickly endear himself to the band staff and to the Band Council. He was friendly, easy-going, unpretentious—especially for a doctor—and interested in everything the band was involved in. He handed out prescriptions for mega-vitamins and iron supplements as though they were valium, and invited patients to go on long walks with him. He spent hours just talking to people. He played with kids and made house calls any time of day or night. He entered the poorest homes on the reserve and never winced. He didn't drink and he ate fish. He performed no operations, choosing to refer people to out-of-town specialists for any serious complaints.

Dr. and Mrs. Rifleman also attended the social functions they were invited to at the Legion, at Dr. Pickup's home, at the nurses' residence, and at the Anglican Minister's house. Slowly but surely, his appointment book began to fill up.

At the band's Christmas party he read a poem he had written and "gave" it to the band:

Words are nothing but empty sounds,
like the pebble's noise in a hollow wood.
So, this Christmas I ask you to wait and watch,
for it is the small daily actions of men which
tell the heart all it needs to know.
Quietly, as you have made me welcome among you,
Quietly, I too will go about my work.
But listen not to the words...
Wait and watch.

Around New Year's, Dr. Rifleman told Wedledi he might have to go away for a while as he thought he may be in some sort of trouble with the American income tax people. He was concerned that if anyone should hear about it they might think less of him. "Don't worry about that!" Wedledi had laughed. "We're fishermen remember!"[1]

On Saturday, January 26, 1980, the R.C.M.P. took Dr. Rifleman out of his clinic in handcuffs and flew him to the Port Hardy lock-up. All through that day and night both Wedledi and the chief, Roy Cranmer, made repeated calls to the jail requesting permission to speak with Dr. Rifleman. They wanted to let him know that whatever it was he'd done, it was O.K.; that no one was angry; that they would get him bail or a lawyer. A few women went to sit with his wife.

The R.C.M.P. would not allow Dr. Rifleman to receive any calls. They told Wedledi that he was charged with impersonating a doctor and practising medicine without a licence. He was wanted on similar charges in the U.S., they said.

"You guys always get the wrong man," Wedledi told the Sergeant cheekily. "It's the doctor *with* the licence you should've arrested!"

In a signed confession to the R.C.M.P. Dr. Rifleman stated that by posing as a doctor he had not intended to make a lot of money. "It just made it possible for me to do what I enjoy doing and that is sort of helping and being a positive part of a community," he said. "I would also like to state that my intention was not to harm anyone or in any way add to the problems of the community in Alert Bay," his statement continued. "I have been treated well by everyone concerned and only wish that I had an opportunity to somehow undo the terrible situation that must follow this flow of events. I would like to make very clear the fact that Dr. Pickup and Mr. Wilkinson [the new administrator at St. George's] had nothing to do with my coming or my leaving...The blame is entirely mine and the consequences that follow are of my own creation....At this point I wish only that I could alter whatever harm I have inflicted on those who have treated me so well."

The following morning the Port Hardy R.C.M.P. called Wedledi. Dr. Rifleman had broken his eye-glasses, wrapped his neck in the cell blanket and slit his jugular vein. He was dead when they checked his cell on Sunday morning. Lying open next to his bunk was a medical book he had asked the police to allow him to keep in his cell. "I love you Claudia" had been scrawled inside the book's cover with coffee.

Mrs. Rifleman quickly left town.

An inquest was held and Wedledi attended and tried to protest the fact that no one had been allowed contact, that Dr. Rifleman hadn't seen a lawyer, and that by the time they found him the R.C.M.P. hadn't checked his cell for over twelve hours.

Wedledi's objections were noted.

Dr. Rifleman turned out to be Roberto Enrique Trujillo, a Chicano born in Albuquerque, New Mexico on January 16, 1933. Both his parents had been alcoholics. His mother had died when he was twelve and his father had disappeared shortly after. When he was fifteen, using forged documents that gave his age as nineteen, he had enlisted in the U.S. Navy. He had spent eleven years in the navy where he trained as a medic and began educating himself in the field of psychology. Following his navy tour, Trujillo had taken a job, under an assumed name, in a New York City child care centre. Within a year he had been appointed director of the centre, but authorities had caught up to him and he had fled to California where he was subsequently arrested and convicted on robbery and assault charges and sentenced to four years. He had continued his self-education in prison, and after being released in 1964 had posed as a physician or psychologist in a number of places in both the U.S.A. and Mexico, under at least eleven aliases.

Trujillo next came to public attention in 1971 when he was arrested in Elgin, Illinois where he had been posing as Dr. Anthony Barton, holder of a Ph.D. in child psychology from the University of California at Berkeley. In Elgin he worked as a child therapist and college lecturer and began building up a private practice. The director of the Larkin Home for Children in Elgin told reporters that "Trujillo was the best child therapist I have ever worked with. I suspect no one as gifted as him will ever come to Elgin again." He added that the children in the home were anxious to know where Trujillo had gone so they could write to him. Students in Trujillo's "Introduction to Group Processes" college course said he was a compassionate man who had "a certain way of touching people." His lawyer described him as an intelligent person with an I.Q. of 145 who "loved people, especially children, and was dedicated to helping them."

Following this arrest, Trujillo was extradited to California to face parole violation charges. He stabbed himself and escaped from the prison hospital where his wounds were being treated. Four years later he was arrested in New York City after he was discovered posing as a child psychologist and running his own private clinic in fashionable Long Island. He escaped custody again and fled to Mexico.

The real Dr. Rifleman, from his home in Wisconsin, told reporters that he had met Trujillo in San Miguel de Allende, Mexico, where Trujillo had been operating a clinic for the poor under the name Dr. Enrique Marti. It was in San Miguel that the real Dr. Rifleman's personal papers, including medical diplomas and photographs, had been stolen. The real Dr. Rifleman described Trujillo as a "likeable, intelligent individual, well-read with a tremendous philosophy on life."

Dr. Pickup took credit for alerting the authorities, claiming he had noticed irregularities in the new doctor's methods. Others said Dr. Pickup had gone looking for "dirt" when it became obvious that the new doctor could be a threat. Dr. Pickup's supporters gloated. The Indians' star doctor had turned out to be a fake.

The Nimpkish Band Council claimed Dr. Rifleman's body when no relatives could be found. The Anglican Church refused to hold services for him as he had committed suicide, so arrangements were made for the preacher at the Indian Pentecostal Church—a local breakaway from the official (White) Pentecostal Church—to hold a service.

The old house that had been converted into a church was filled to capacity on the day of the funeral. Over 200 people listened as the lay preacher quickly dealt with Rifleman's criminal record and suicide by quoting from the Bible: "Let the man who has not sinned, let that man cast the first stone."

The funeral procession wound its way up the hill to the new Indian graveyard. The people who twelve months previously had been knocking on doors tentatively asking people to sign a petition for better medical care trudged along behind the old hearse: little groups of three or four people leaning weakly on each other for support. Some weren't on speaking terms with others any more. Pearl and Wedledi were leaving their jobs at the band office after a dispute with the Band Council, and most of us on the Education Committee were making plans to move out of town for a while.

Band Councillor Chris Cook delivered a eulogy at the graveside:

> He may not have been a real doctor but at least he has shown us
> the kind of treatment we have a right to expect. He came and helped
> us in our distress. We don't condemn this man. He was our friend.

We stood silently as the coffin was lowered into the ground, tears streaming down our cheeks. Inside we were numb. We felt no strength, no force—not even anger. We were hardly conscious of crying any more. Our tears had taken on a life of their own and came and went as they pleased.

Dr. Rifleman used to say that if he died in Alert Bay, he wanted to be buried in the Indian cemetery on the hill, overlooking the water and the mountains. That is where we laid his body to rest. His grave is marked by a small wooden cross which bears the inscription: DOCTOR ROBERT RIFLEMAN.

" 'Cause that's how we knew him," Wedledi said.

NOTES:

[1]Fishermen are classified as self-employed and income tax is not deducted at source. As a rule, fishermen are notoriously hard to collect income tax from and some Indian fishermen still feel that they were unfairly tricked into paying income tax during the Second World War. Consequently, playing cat and mouse with Revenue Canada until the inevitable, inescapable blue "garnishee" notice arrives is sort of a local sport.

CHAPTER 11

The Inquiry

But the rock can never triumph
And the egg it dare not rot

For if the egg is shattered
Then splattered is the rock!

Alert Bay,
March, 1980

On March 3, 1980, the Government of Canada Inquiry into Indian Health and Health Care in Alert Bay, B.C. opened in the gymnasium of the old residential school, under Commissioner Dr. Gary Goldthorpe, a man experienced in the field of Indian health, a former Zone Director for Medical Services in the Sioux Lookout region of Ontario, and well-respected by Indian groups with whom he worked in Eastern Canada. Michael Jackson had arrived two weeks earlier to co-ordinate the preparations for the inquiry. Although the group who had started everything had shattered into splinters, once again people put aside their disputes. Once again, long days and nights were spent compiling briefs, documenting cases, typing, photocopying, living on coffee and sandwiches. Once again, Kwakwaka'wakw from Alert Bay and surrounding villages, old and young, filled the gym in the old residential school.

Dr. Goldthorpe set out the terms of reference for the Inquiry:

The World Health Organization has defined health as not just the absence of disease or disability but a state of total physical, mental and social well-being....I expect to be drawing these connections in our meetings and if this Commission reaches conclusions that are outside the area of jurisdiction of the Minister of National Health and Welfare Canada, I expect that the conclusions and recommendations will be passed on to the other appropriate agencies.

Following Dr. Goldthorpe's opening address, Chief Roy Cranmer set out the following objectives on behalf of the Nimpkish Band Council:

This Inquiry is something for which we have fought for over a year...We wish to know why is our rate of hospitalization and our death rate so high? And why is our life expectancy so low? Why is our survival threatened? What is the quality of our health care services? Why have so many of our people lost confidence in the health care we have been receiving?

We hope to demonstrate through our presentation this week, that the problems that face us go far beyond the practices of one local doctor. They date back one hundred years to the attitude and state of mind that characterizes non-Indian behaviour towards Indians...

A representative of the elders of the Native community, Mr. Jack Peters, was the next to address the gathering:

We have come because we have been invited by this person, to make understood the way we did things when we were growing up, all of us people....Now have come the children, the new children of today. Our law has changed, we who are Indians. I have let go from my hands that which I would have looked after.... Alcohol does not belong to us. It belongs to you, you white people, when you came here, to make money from our people. You made your money and a beer parlour was built. Young people went into this place. I was among them. Now I have stopped. I stopped drinking more than ten years ago, because I saw that it meant nothing....

Now I hope what you are speaking of turns out well, that you are asking us to speak of things, including early medicines and the business of drinking....You can see what is the right way to make this stop. You have all gone to school. We were told, 'Whoever does not go to school, will come to no good.' So, what of today? You are supposed to see the good way to be, at the present time. The Bible was brought to our land, for us to obey. You have been told, you children of to-day...I have sat in church, I have spoken in church, helping those who want help. That is the only way it will be worked out, that it will stop—to depend on Him who created us.

You know of the great flood—would we have returned here as men, if the early people did not believe and save themselves to come back to this land? And we are still here on this land. We are still here on this land. Some people say we near to disaster. Yes, we will have disaster if the white people fight [again]...But we do not fight any more, we who are Indians. I was included with those who went to fight the last time. I signed my name to kill Germans, but I did not cross the water, because it was over...Many of our people were taken to go to fight... So that you can see...Look at what I have to say.

What the young people do is powerfully bad. They do everything—smoking bad tobacco, swallowing pills. These things do not belong to us, we who are Indians....When we still live in our village, we were threatened that if we didn't move to a place with a school, we would not become better, so we came here and what good has it done us? Hardly any of us work, although there is a school here.

Now, look at today—how have they improved? None.

There is no way in which we do not suffer now, children. People all over the world suffer now, I know, because of change in our ways. That is all I have.

Wedledi Speck expressed the feelings of many who had spent the preceeding fifteen months on the front lines of this particular battleground:

I am only participating in this Inquiry because it is important to let the Government of Canada and its people know what they have done and are doing to our people. I hope to bring to light enough evidence to persuade yourself, Mr. Commissioner, and some of our own people, and the Canadian people, that *racism* was the biggest factor that forced a change in our way of life and still remains a factor in preventing our leaders from taking charge of our lives again...

I want to insure people that Indians are human beings, are capable of ruling our own lives as did our forefathers and do not need the social do-gooder attitude that perpetuates racism.

The first day of public hearings was devoted to presentations on aboriginal medicines by the old people, who were introduced by their interpreters, Bob Joseph and Gloria Cranmer Webster.

Bob:

    To my immediate right is Billy Sandy Willie from Tsawataineuk... He's 91 years old. Next to him is Jack Peters of the Tenakteuk. He doesn't know his exact age but he knows he's over 80 years old. This is Jane Willie. She's over 80 years old. And the young lady in the white hair is Granny Axu. She's 91. Next here is Mrs. Agnes Cranmer. She's 72 and next to her is Emma Beans. She didn't want to tell us her age, but we finally got it out of her. She's 73. Mrs. Ethel Alfred next to her is just a kid. She's 69.

The old people began to speak among themselves in Kwa'kwala while Gloria and Bob hastily scribbled notes, asked questions and translated for the audience and the Commissioner.

Gloria:

    Axu says there were very few diseases....That in the old days, a lot of people bathed in real ice cold water and helped to build their resistance...now, she says, everybody gets a little bit of a chill and they all get colds and get sick....Mrs. Alfred said one of the illnesses of early people was what is now known as arthritis and that the treatment for that was a mixture of yellow cedar. It was mixed and heated. The patient would be covered completely with these various plants in a container and the steam from this would be allowed to cover them underneath this blanket, and that that was a treatment that worked well for what we now know as arthritis....For toothaches hadzapame' (yarrow) was chewed. It took away the pain and the swelling....Tł'i'na is the oil rendered from oolichans and is used primarily as a food but also it was used as a medicine in earlier times. During flu epidemics, many people owed their survival to drinking the oolichan oil....The treatment for cuts, very bad cuts was to take a snail, cut it open and lay it on the cut and it was left on the cut until it had dried up.

Charlie Matilipi (from the audience):

    Yes. I was cured from that...Anybody squashes snail now...not my friend!

Ethel Alfred:

    I had experience with that snail too. I cut my foot when I was about eleven, so we were all alone at Village Island and I had it put on my foot and I never came to see the doctor and it was healed in about a couple of weeks....With one of my boys you know, when he was a baby...he had no skin on his buttocks. It just was all red. The skin was so red and I had to take him to the doctor so many times and nothing did anything for him you know. So my mom went in the woods and got some alder bark and she scrubbed alder bark and put boiling water over it and let it stand for overnight and she just took the water out and then she told me, when I bathed my baby just put a cupful of that alder water on him and so I used to just let it dry on him. In a week's time, he was all better, never had it ever since....Another experience I have is my sister-in-law had eczema so bad she couldn't even bend her fingers. She had a baby at that time and she was going to Rivers Inlet with my brother so my mother said I'll go and get you some alder. So she told her what to do...just soak your hands in it and just take it out and let it dry and my sister-in-law said she only did that for about ten days and she went filling cans in the cannery after that. Her hands were all cured. So she never had it back...So I really have great faith in our medicines....

Bob:

All the old people recall many many old people reaching ripe old ages. There were so many more old people in the villages than there are now....They did mention that there was a high infant mortality rate, that lots of babies did die in the old days, but once having survived, I guess the initial stages, you lived to be very old....I asked the old people about alcoholism in the early days. They said alcoholism didn't come until the white man came through. It kind of became a tradition with fishermen to celebrate the catch and it just went from bad to worse.

Commissioner Goldthorpe:

I would like to know from the older people if they have any ideas what is likely to help us with this problem?

Gloria:

Axu feels that when potlatches were outlawed, our people lost a kind of control that the older people had had over the younger people. It was a time for instructing the young people in proper behaviour....Gwanti'lakw says when she was growing up, that people of her age never saw their parents drinking in their homes. It just wasn't done and that now when children are fifteen and sixteen, they think that they are grown up to drink and carry on in that fashion....

Commissioner:

Can you ask the older people why Indian medicines are not used any more?

Gloria:

There were a lot of medicine men earlier....every village had their own. The last one was from New Vancouver and I remember him when I was a child. A lot of white people went to him too, this man from New Vancouver.

Bob:

Granny Axu says that Indian medicines are still used and up until very recently they had been using them more....But the main reason for a shift away from Indian medicine was that they had been encouraged by doctors and other professionals that this new medicine was, I suppose, superior and they put their faith in that and kind of drifted away from native medicine. And too that there was so many new sicknesses when the white man came through that maybe their medicines weren't ready for.

Gloria:

In our discussions with our older people, one of the points they made is that for them, health meant "strength," łaxwe'." Their knowledge of traditional medicines and their uses was to ensure that strength....It is difficult to talk only of traditional medical practices among our people. This is a white man's way of looking at things— so that now we have dental health, mental health and all sorts of other categories and rarely is a patient looked at as a total human being. The "strength" our old people refer to was the health of the whole person....Whatever problems we faced in the old days were problems created within our own communities, and over centuries, these communities had worked out solutions to these problems....

We know from our discussions with the old people that the matter of health or "strength" was the concern of all people in the community. Children learned from their parents and grandparents the proper observances to maintain strength. They learned to identify a wide variety of plant materials and learned how to use these as effective medicines and as food. These learning experiences had continued in the same way for generations, until the white people came. When children began being taken away from parents and placed in missionary schools, this traditional kind of learning decreased, but there was not a corresponding growth of knowledge of white man's medicine at the same time.

Indian people were discouraged from using traditional medicines. In fact, some of the old people have told us that they were told these were poisonous. What happened to our people happened elsewhere in the world, where colonizers moved in. Outsiders came to an area unknown to them and began imposing their own standards on the aboriginal peoples. At no time was there an effort on the part of the outsiders to understand...or to blend the old with the new in a way that would least take away the strength of the native people. We were colonized by white people who were convinced that whatever practices they saw among us, because they were different, had to be inferior, uncivilized, heathen. It was ethnocentricity at its most destructive level....

If we think of health as strength, we were rapidly becoming an unhealthy people, unable to oppose the changes taking place in our lives. We were losing our strength in all areas....

We are no longer as vulnerable as we were. Gradually, we are regaining our strength and becoming healthy again.

This Inquiry must be one way of demonstrating to the larger community that we must make decisions that affect our lives and our strength. For ourselves, this Inquiry must demonstrate that no one *gives* you strength. Each of us must build this within ourselves because no matter what this Inquiry accomplishes in terms of improving health care services to our people, we have our own work to do if we are to survive as a people of strength.

These sessions were followed by presentations on behalf of the Band and District Councils, which documented the economic history of the Kwakwaka'wakw—particulary in relation to the declining fishing industry.

Chief Basil Ambers:
....One by one, the villages throughout this area have been deserted. No longer could the old ways of food collection be employed, for devastation of the environment required further travel afield to obtain these staple food items....It is not therefore surprising that there was an attendant decline in the feeling of economic and social well-being, and thus physical health.

We are becoming a landlocked people on this Coast! ...In order to have pride, you've got to have economic well-being as well as the spiritual well-being. Without any involvement in any industry whatsoever, then really there is no way that you can ever hold your head up, so every time you get a welfare cheque or whatever it is—down to the beer parlour or straight into the liquor store....

In closing, Mr. Commissioner, I would like to state once more that I feel very strongly....I become very angry when I realize that other people will not allow us to participate in the very things that affect us and in a matter such as health...I feel so strongly about that that I sometimes feel like I look at people and almost lose the ability to speak.

Ernest Willie, of the Kwakiutl District Council, spoke about growing up in his village and about what he had learned about life and about Kwakwaka'wakw ways from the old people. He also talked about change, and about his experiences in residential school:

> Our parents waited in anger, bewilderment for that little brown envelope with the little window on it that was addressed to them from the Department of Indian Affairs, and they would open it with hesitation to find the names of their children that were required to report here at the St. Michael's School, Alert Bay, that particular September.
>
> I spent eight years here and in those eight years, I could say that I am both a victim and a product of a school system that the Church of England introduced to this country. Why was my people so weak-kneed in such a short time? That's what I wondered. How come the encroachment upon them as a people, us people, why did it deteriorate so fast? Used to be here for ten months of the year, and that—I'm remembering—there used to be two lines of chairs in that hallway and if our parents happened to be in town, they came to visit us, but there was always a staff member standing there, making sure that they didn't speak 'that language.' I used to wonder about it and even as a big kid, because I didn't go to school until I was ten...Crying myself to sleep every night. Why? No longer was there any pride that could well from within, so you strive to be....
>
> The one year I did that in this school. I decided that the conformity to St. Michael's School was the optimum and that was when I was fourteen. I learned how to speak English. I used to go out in those woods back there and I take a reader and it was called 'High Roads Reader' and I would go and read to all the trees and anything that looked like it could listen to me. You know how trees go, you know, the bows go like this and they sort of look like, you know, they are listening to you and say 'Go Ahead.' I used to look at, for instance, I remember looking at and admiring someone like King George VI, I guess it was, and his brother who abdicated that throne. Maybe I don't have my history right? But I remember seeing those men and they were men of honour and they had a presence about them that was unshakeable. Now I look at those guys—well, guys like that— and I think, that was our chiefs before. They were men like that. But then I didn't think about that like that, I just kind of looked at King George...Like that's the way to be, you know.

Next, presentations were made on the history of band administration and relationships with the Department of Indian Affairs regarding Indian takeovers of DIA programs, lack of funding, red tape, incompetent advisors, etc. The documentation presented was thorough, and Wedledi expressed the reality beyond the facts and figures:

> It's a lot harder to point out the attitude that I speak of, but it is there. The only difference is that the Department of Indian Affairs personnel no longer write openly about how they feel. You have to watch the action and see it. You have to be there...you have to experience the frustration at the Kwakiutl District Council, at the Band Councils, ...the frustration...that they go through....

Next came testimony from those who had submitted affidavits, letters or statements of complaint to the various authorities such as the College of Physicians and Surgeons during the past year. Once again, the community laid open its wounds and set down in the public record their experiences with Dr. Pickup, with the hospital, with the federal Indian health service. This session was opened by a statement from Renee Smith's family, read by her aunt, Elizabeth:

> We wanted to see justice done in the death of my niece. That process that we felt was a just search for the truth was extremely painful for myself and other members of my family...We believed that our complaints and demands for solution could be brought about through regular channels...We believed that the appropriate action would be taken to make sure that other people would not suffer the fate of my niece...We have suffered many indignities and disappointments...It has been suggested over and over again that we are not telling the truth...Meanwhile, an imposter comes to practice medicine in Alert Bay, sanctioned by this same body whose only interest appears to be protecting its own. Nevertheless, the so-called Doctor Rifleman displayed a sympathy and sensitivity far beyond that of our long-term resident doctor. At least he was a person that really cared and tried within his limited knowledge to help, for which he's accepted in the end.
>
> As we relive the pain and the loss of Renee at your Inquiry now, will it be another exercise in futility of which your findings and recommendations will have no bearing? Will other children die needlessly? Will other Indians die of neglect or error, ignorance or indifference and if they do, will anybody care?...That's the kind of stuff we have had to go through...Renee should not have died in vain...Thank you.

Two more of Renee's aunts, Eva Cook and Vera Cranmer, talked about their aunt, Louisa James',[1] death.

Eva:

One night in the hospital, after her operation, when she did sleep, Doctor Pickup walked in and walked over to her bed and poked her in her stomach where she was lying...It was so swollen...He poked her and woke her up and asked her how she was feeling. Louisa got mad and she swore at him and told him to get out because he was drunk...I kept saying 'Doctor Pickup, I want Louisa to be brought to Vancouver. There's something wrong with her.' He said 'No. It costs too much money. You people don't have that kind of money to take her down.' I said 'Doctor Pickup', I says, 'I come from a big family' I said. 'Money is no problem. We can all get our money together and send her away.' But no, he wouldn't let her go.

So Mr. Commissioner, I feel that something has to be done. I feel very strongly about this.

Vera sobbed as she spoke:

We...our people look after our own. When our people die, we dress them ourselves. This thing with morticians is just a new thing...The day of Auntie Louisa's funeral, we couldn't allow anyone to see her...the condition she was in...

I'd like to see justice done here. We've all suffered through it so much. We don't want to see it happen again. If only this had happened ...what we're doing here today before...when we lost...Maybe we would have still had some of our loved ones with us now....

Thank you, Mr. Commissioner.

Often with great embarrassment, people told their stories. Some asked other people to present their statements for them. One of the chiefs read his daughter's letter:

I was born in Alert Bay and have spent most of my life here.

Up until about two years ago my relationship with Dr. Pickup was on a friendly basis although I did not go to him for major medical problems.

Last year I went in to get a salpinogram test done. After the test was over he informed me that one fallopian tube was blocked completely but the other was open. When I tried to question him further on the implications of the results he told me again the results and to make a further appointment with him if I wished to know further. Then he immediately left me there in the office.

A couple of weeks later I was sitting in the local bar and Dr. H. J. Pickup walked in and joined me. At this point, after he appeared to have consumed a fair amount of alcohol, he turned the conversation

242

over to my tests and told me that I could not have children. He said he had done all the testing he could do for me, which he summarized by saying words to the effect that he felt it was good that I could not have children because he didn't think I should. At this point I don't think it is necessary for me to say how I felt. My brother was sitting with Dr. Pickup and I and heard the conversation and will verify it if necessary.

It was a very unprofessional and unethical move on his part and caused me a great deal of anguish. Later, after making a further investigation of my test results in Vancouver I found out that this test alone is only one of the very first tests done when trying to determine whether or not women can have children and that the results of a salpingogram are not conclusive without further testing.

For two full days people continued to come forward. The prepared agenda quickly became meaningless and evening sessions were scheduled so that everyone who wished to could have an opportunity to speak:

Hello Mr. Commissioner. My name is Ann[2] and I've lived in Alert Bay all of my life. During the summer of 1975—I was seventeen years old—I was in a position where I had to help a friend go to the hospital. I suspected he was suffering from a drug overdose. He was very blue. He was, you know, he could hardly breathe. When we got to the hospital, two nurses immediately came to attend to this person. They started panicking, they didn't know how to deal with the situation. They couldn't even get the oxygen tank going....Dr. Pickup arrived and asked me, you know, what was going on and I said I didn't know, he was the doctor. I just, you know, the person was ill and I thought this was where I was supposed to bring him. He asked me if I was certain that it was a drug overdose and I said well, all I knew was that in town, there was a lot of talk about methadone going around.

Dr. Pickup flipped out at this point and started to shout and scream at me about he was the only doctor north of Campbell River that provided methadone for heroin treatment and that obviously if this person had it, it had to have come from one of his patients. I said "I don't know, you're the doctor...I don't know any of these people." He said he didn't want to save this person, it was a waste of his time, it was about ten o'clock in the evening and he had had to come from home and he just kept yelling at me and then he called the police and they started to carry on at me.

Meanwhile, nobody was...the only thing he had done for the person was to give him oxygen. Then they took him in the operating room and did whatever was required. I was sitting in the waiting room and

Dr. Pickup came out and told me very angrily that if it ever happened again, not to bother coming back. He said that he was not going to bother saving people who were going to deliberately kill themselves. I said he had no right to say that. He didn't know if the person deliberately took an overdose and he was the only doctor so I was very upset that he would say he wouldn't save someone. The police kept questioning me and I just said you're talking to the wrong person. I just brought this person here because he was unconscious.

Also I'd like to say about other doctors....I became very ill one night in 1978 with pains in my abdomen. I went to the hospital and Pickup was the only one there. He examined me and said well, it isn't appendicitis but you stay in the hospital here and we'll see what's the matter. I said no, I'm not going to do that. I want to go to Vancouver because I'm still in pain. Dr. Pickup became very angry and was yelling at me that the doctors in Vancouver couldn't do anything for me that he couldn't do and I just said it's a matter of opinion and it's my right. I'm leaving.

So I got to Vancouver and they put me in the hospital and the doctor comes around and he takes my history and he says "Oh, you're from Alert Bay. Is that drunk doctor still there?" I got angry. I was really mad. I said why should I have to fly to Vancouver to hear you tell me that the doctor in my home town is a drunk and you just laugh about it. He just said "Well, you know, there's nothing you can do about it. He's given a lot of good service over the years." I've gone to other doctors and it's always the same. They're always interested that you come from Alert Bay and they all know about him but then they just keep quiet when they see that you don't think it's a joke.

All these things are written in an affidavit that I submitted when we were trying to petition for this Inquiry and I hope that somebody's going to listen to us finally and accept it. Thank you.

Witness after witness spoke to the assembly. Many broke down and couldn't finish their presentations. Friends and relatives stood and filled in for them. Once again, the Indian community sat and listened and cried and watched the Commissioner. Once again, the media recounted the horrors to the world. The non-Indian community was conspicuous by its absence.

Mayor Gilbert Popovich, however, who along with two aldermen who were recent arrivals in town, had been dropping in on the hearings during his time off from cab-driving, made a presentation on behalf of the Municipal Council.

Mayor Popovich read the brief his council had just submitted to the B.C. Hospitals Association and the B.C. Ministry of Health. It outlined the minimum health facilities and medical staffing the council felt was necessary for Alert Bay:

(1) 25 bed hospital

(2) an advanced laboratory

(3) two full-time physicians with separate practices

(4) professional drug and alcohol counsellors.

A Chief from one of the villages asked:

I'd like to ask the Mayor and the people that put that submission together, why is it that there is nothing in there for preventative medicine?

The Mayor replied:

We made mention about the fact that there are sociological problems and the only way to solve those is to have the type of counselling and educational programs and preventive work necessary to overcome it.

Chief Basil Ambers:

Now, the health needs of this area are very important to everybody in this area, but it's very indicative that there's very few from the other end of town here. It says volumes to me anyway—that the only thing that the Honourable Mayor from the other end of town had to say to this gathering here was a plea for support for his 25-bed hospital....

Chief Roy Cranmer:

It's just you guys' attitude about this thing...yours...the Hospital Board's, the regional board, the provincial government, right up to the line, you know. I mean nobody is listening to us....I mean, it's typical that you guys, if you need us, you come and see us...

I think the picture that keeps developing here is that Indian statistics are always being used by the non-Indian groups to procure funds from the Feds and I think what we're trying to say is that it's about time Indian statistics are used by Indians, for their own benefit...

The Mayor:

Well...I do try......

The Nimpkish Band's head alcohol and drug counsellor agreed with the Mayor that working together would be a better solution:

I was fortunate enough to have lived on this Reserve when our people were still living as Indians, proud and independent, caring people who worked together, lived together and cared about one another. There

245

was very little drinking and children were cared for.

This is not to say that they are not cared for today, we have very many fine people who do not fall into this category, but we have many people who have a problem of alcoholism. Drinking is not an Indian way of life. We have not had centuries to adapt to drinking, so as a result, we become alcoholics sooner than non-Indians. This is a sad fact. Alcoholism is the cause of at least 99% of all the deaths on this Reserve, directly or indirectly. For example, drowning or, lately, car accidents.

Alcohol is destroying our people, our way of life, our Indian culture and self-respect. The thing that alarms me most as an alcohol counsellor is our under-age people's easy access to alcohol. People do not seem to fear any consequences for supplying and they do get away with it.

I attend court once a month, and I have never heard anyone being prosecuted for supplying to minors. There was a time when illegal selling of alcohol, namely bootlegging, happened only in the municipality, and now we have some of our own people doing this vulturous and horrendous deed. Words cannot express adequately how I feel towards these people who are preying for financial gain on the unfortunate people's addiction to alcohol.

And as if this is not enough, we also have on the scene, prescription drugs and street drugs destroying our people. This is the cause of all the crimes our young people commit since marijuana and acid are expensive to acquire and these young people are unemployed, they resort to crime.

I feel that working together we could achieve some positive results. If we remain divided, it will take longer to resolve this very very sad problem. I feel that as a solution to this problem there needs to be a closer working relationship with the R.C.M.P., Municipal Council, Nimpkish Band Council, and all resource people in Alert Bay, with no strings attached on either side.

We should be looking forward to attending the weddings of our young people. Unfortunately, we will be attending the funerals of some of them.

By the fourth day, the audience, including those of us who had sworn we were not going to participate at all, was ready to explode. Some had been waiting for this inquiry for over a year. Most had been waiting for it all their lives.

The Zone Director for Medical Services, Dr. Mary Habgood, took the stand and outlined all the personnel employed by, and the services performed by, her department: Public Health Nurses, Dental Therapists, Alcohol Counsellors, Psychologists, Health Educators, Nutritionists, Community Health Representatives, Environmental Health Officers provide prosthetics including glasses, dentures and wheelchairs; pre-natal and post-natal counselling; in-school examinations for ear disease, vision defects, dental disease and infestations such as nits and scabies and immunization programs including regular X-rays for communicable diseases, particularly T.B. and hepatitis. Dr. Habgood agreed, however, that a more "holistic" approach was needed:

> I think solution of some of these problems, you know, the continual put-downs, the poor economic conditions and unemployment and the bureaucratic hassles will do much to reduce the dependence on alcohol, and then the related medical environment conditions that are causing sickness and death. The size of the problem has been very well documented by the Nimpkish Band.

A band member later responded to this impressive list with the following anecdote:

> I would like to mention something in terms of Medical Services in that I had an experience with Medical Services here with my daughter who was having ear problems...
> You, as a mother, walk into the room with your child and there's usually Dr. Pickup, the specialist, the Health Nurse and the Community Health Representative. At that time, we had another doctor here who was also in attendance. I took my little girl in and she was sat down and examined. The doctors discussed in highly technical terms what they considered wrong with her; then they relayed that to the Health Nurse. The Health Nurse told the CHR and the CHR took me outside and said "Right, we can get her a bed in the Children's Hospital for such and such a date. She's got _____," which was a long technical term which I didn't understand. I said no. I said I have no reason to trust this doctor. I've never seen him before. He doesn't even have the decency to talk to me. Why on earth should I trust him to operate on my child? I said I want a second opinion. She said well that's very unusual. I said I don't care, I'll make arrangements myself. I called my sister's doctor in Vancouver and asked for a referral and made an appointment for my daughter to see another specialist. I kept, you know, the hospital arrangements that they had made and I simply said I wanted another opinion before I was going to allow her to have any kind of operation.
> When I went to the Health Centre — the hospital appointment was for a Monday, the appointment I made with the specialist of my own choice was on a Friday. I went down to the Health Centre on Wednesday to get a travel warrant to take my daughter to the hospital, to Vancouver for these appointments, and was told the travel warrant

247

would only be issued as of Sunday, the night before the appointment on Monday.

I explained that I had made an appointment with a specialist in order to get a second opinion and that that appointment was on Friday and I was told by the Nurse that Medical Services is not in the habit of paying for people to spend weekends in Vancouver. I got very angry because, like they were accusing me of using my daughter's ear problem to go partying in Vancouver or something! You just have to see the way they look at people, like they can hardly control the looks on their faces sometimes.

Vera Robinson questioned the Zone Director for Medical Services on her responsibility in the "Pickup business." Had she received complaints from her staff? Yes. For how long? Three or four years. (But, she had, she admitted later, warned a health nurse about the doctor's drinking habits *seven* years ago.) Had she had complaints from the Nimpkish Band Council? "Yes, I had had complaints from the Band Office of rudeness and of lack of referral and of a physician attending on occasions to see patients drunk," Dr. Habgood replied.

Vera:

As a member of the College of Physicians and Surgeons, did you voice those concerns to your registration body?[3]

Dr. Habgood:

No. I advised the people who had the complaints that they should be directed personally by them to the College....I think it was my place to help people do something about it.

A band member pursued this line of questioning.

Kelly:

In your opinion...the basis for this inquiry is inadequate medical services being provided to Indian people. What is your opinion of that position and your responsibility as an employee of Medical Services and as a human being who has been involved in Indian health for so long?

Dr. Habgood:

I'm just not quite sure of your question. I think that there is a need for an Inquiry. There's a need for discussion of the whole gamut of medical services and there is certainly some room for improvement....

Kelly:

So within the guidelines that you have for your job, you think that you're doing an adequate job....So how has all this changed anything?

Dr. Habgood:

I think we've all learned a lot from this situation...and I certainly think that if I receive the kinds of complaints that I did say from the Band Council before, I would have—in future—I would be far more forthcoming in trying to help them get to the proper authorities...I think the most important thing is that we are all far more sensitive to complaints...

Chief Basil Ambers:

Sensitivity is very nice, Doctor, but our people are dying!

A middle-aged woman, now resident in Victoria, asked for a spot on the agenda:

Thank you Mr. Commissioner. For your information—everybody else here knows who I am—I am a member of the mighty Kwaguitl Nation.

For years and years...Every sports day in June, our people here put on dances, brought out their sacred costumes and dance to raise money for this hospital here. People came from the inlets partly in their canoes, partly in gas boats, broken down old boats sometime, to bring their treasured masks and things to dance. It is surely time, Mr. Commissioner that this was looked into. Our chiefs are never listened to. We're always pushed aside. I am very shaken up about what's been going on so I don't beg. I demand that a real inquiry is made here in Alert Bay.

Last Thursday, we were phoned that my nephew had been drowned and we rushed up here, of course, and then they told us that a day later his body was found and—to my untrained thoughts—it was just a simple case of drowning. But when we got up here...the man in charge told us that we couldn't bury Sam because they had sent his body to Vancouver. The family was never asked if they wanted an autopsy, they were just told it had to be done. So then we think it wasn't just a common drowning. So they took his body down Sunday night and they assured us he would be—the body would be—back Monday and we could have the funeral on Tuesday.

Well, Tuesday came along and they told us that the body had been inadvertently dropped off at Port Hardy and that when the guy went to get it, they told him the body was dropped off in Campbell River. What kind of bungling is that that my people have to endure? This always happens in Alert Bay and this is not an isolated case. I have seen this happen because unfortunately, every time I visit my people up here, it is because one of my loved ones had died and there's always this unnecessary delays, unnecessary bungling and now that the autopsies are performed, we have never ever been told what their findings are. Surely we are not that naive and trusting that we have to take the white man's word for everything that happens to us. We are intelligent enough, and always have been from the beginning of time, to rule our own destiny.

You know, the kid wasn't brought up here until Wednesday night by the time they found his body. We are not even given any dignity in death any more. If he had come back when they said he was going to come back we would have been able to dress him. It is a tradition with my people that we like to dress our own. As it was, they put him in a plastic bag and forbid us; the man came to the house about ten o'clock that night and told us you are not to open the casket. (Thank God you people paid for a sealed casket, Your Honour!)

What kind of bullshit is that? (Pardon me, Your Honour, but that's exactly how I feel!)

And his mother and father…it is a custom of our people to dress their people and lay them out so that the people can come and pay their final respects. This boy was 31 years old in the prime of his manhood. Couldn't he have left this world in some sort of dignity, instead of being shoved around by the R.C.M.P. and the Medical Board?

Next on the hot seat was Duncan Clarke, Special Assistant to the B.C. Regional Director of the Department of Indian Affairs and Northern Development, whose presentation, like that of the Zone Director of Medical Services, outlined the legislative responsibility of the D.I.A.N.D. and its relationship to both the Indian Health Services Division of National Health and Welfare Canada and to the provincial government in terms of health care to on-reserve Indians. Like the Zone Director, the Assistant Regional Director's statement listed service after service and program after program each of which had a vast sum of money attached to it. The audience was not impressed.

Chief Basil Ambers:
    Since some of the Bands have taken over their own administration over the past, I'd say, eight, nine years within this District, why has the DIA Campbell River District Office more than tripled their staff when supposedly the band has taken over their administration, taken over some of those jobs? We've been asking that question for three years now and we still haven't got an answer.

Duncan Clarke:

It just doesn't work that way. It is recognized, and it is recognized anywhere, that in turning programs over to Indian communities, to Band Councils, that it's going to cost more, not less, for this transition period....

Chief Basil Ambers:

Thanks. For nothing....

Duncan Clarke:

I was not in any way attempting to defend the Department this morning. It was more a case of laying it on the line and saying that this is the way it is, this is the reality of the situation. I'm not defending the Department, when we recognize paternalism and all the damage that it has done over the years. I do say, however, that in recognizing how wrong the situation has been, this Department has gone out of its way to try to change the direction of its own efforts and in the '60s, there was introduced a Community Development Program...This was the beginning, this was the push towards getting Indian people able to speak up and speak out and the Department started to listen. You see, I'm not defending anything. The Department took one long time to start listening, but they are listening....

Chief Basil Ambers:

I don't quite believe you. I'll be as blunt as that. I call that a lie...that you are changing...and I want it to go down on record so that the rest of the people can realize that the things you are saying to me is ridiculous. The only time we ever see anybody with any real authority is when we make enough noise....

Duncan Clarke:

These are the kinds of things that I look forward to when I come to a meeting like this. I am here to listen and I will take both those..you know...after the meeting, we can get together and...the detail...and you will get an answer...Anything I hear, the R.D. will hear. O.K.? ...Meaningful consultation is the name of the game.

At this point, Bob Joseph, a Kwakwaka'wakw man in his forties who had worked for the D.I.A.N.D. for many years intervened.

It always seems such a futile exercise to go through this kind of exercise where we don't really have the answers, you know, and I imagine, well, I don't imagine—I know—it's frustrating when somebody asks a question and we don't have an answer for it and may never have the answer because of our system and structure. While the Department sees itself only in the light of a supportive and helping role, the Indian people see it as a domineering and controlling force. While the Department demands what they feel is good administrative practice and procedure, the Indians see it as infringement and enforcement.

It's so futile to be here, sitting here and seeing Duncan getting run through the wringer when Duncan doesn't have any answers and probably after to-day, he won't have any. He can go back and articulate some of the various specific kinds of questions that were raised, but we will still be here 100 years from now....if we don't dismantle this bureaucracy...

Some people that are in the Department shouldn't be there to begin with because of some of their attitudes. Some of them think that we are just a bunch of welfare bums, you know, and that we are taking this government for a ride and living off public expense and some do think that way and that infringes on the kind of flexibility that policy-makers try to keep inherent in some of the policies...

We will be a little bit older but we will be...same exercise...still here with the same problems because... like everybody has been saying, there is too much external forces trying to shape your mind and that's what it's all about, you know, because that's what this whole Department does and government does and just Canadians in general do. They try to tell you as Indian people that you're different, you know, that your difference is not good and you're not like them. You're never going to amount to a hill of beans, you know. Everything that they do and tell you...health nurses, policemen, it doesn't matter who it is. Every day somebody tells you're different and it's not very good. You better shape up or you're going to be shipped out—you know...

And this entire and devastating process has been termed a conflict of values....This conflict should have taught us something. It should have taught us that Indian people have never surrendered nor capitulated totally.

At the same time, you're probably wondering, well why am I working for this Department after all this criticism of it. Well, it's just because I know it's going to be around for sometime and that for many Indian people and Indian bands, it's still a reality, one that they don't particularly like and that they'd like to see changed, you know, and I want to try to help it to facilitate, maybe, some of those very limited kinds of change.

A young man in the audience jumped up:

You are talking about control over funds. It's control over funds, right. It's control over individuals like me, too...and here you are, both of you, confused! You don't know what's happening. 100 years later, I'll be dead...

Vera Robinson, former Indian Health Nurse and now Nimpkish Band Alcohol Counsellor addressed the inquiry:

A gentleman said 2000 years ago, the unexamined life is not worth living. I think that obviously is a good idea or else it wouldn't have stood the test of time. I commend the Nimpkish Band for examining their lives. Health is not an easy subject. If I am challenged about health, that makes me take a deep breath because straight away, what did I do wrong? Years ago, what did—how come I didn't look after myself? It's not an easy task. I commend everybody that's come forward, that's going to come forward to have their life examined....

As an Indian Health Nurse working different areas, it's easy to see where those government dollars go; they go to look after the white person, they go to look after the Indian Health Nurse coming into a town; it's her house that's wired, it's her house that's got water.... Indian people don't have input into those decisions. They don't have the power and they don't get the running water....

Looking at myself as an Indian Health Nurse, it's very easy to do a job when you're not accountable to the people you're serving....I'm accountable to the Nimpkish Band...I appreciate that accountability because like I know where I'm at....If the present nurse was accountable she would be here too. She's accountable to her bureaucracy so she's not here at this hearing. She's probably a very nice lady, they are probably all decent human beings, but if they're not accountable to the people they're working for, you don't get service.

\ The Union of British Columbia Indian Chiefs and the National Indian Brotherhood made presentations which attested to the fact that the complaints about the delivery of health care being voiced in Alert Bay could be heard in Indian communities from one end of the country to the other, and emphasized the interconnectedness of health and political, social, cultural and economic well-being in general.

We believe this inquiry will support our claims for Indian control, but while this develops, we expect some serious changes in the attitudes of those providing our health care....We need to be more and more involved as shown by the Nimpkish Band in their struggle to get to where they are at today. It hasn't come easy. They have had to fight and we are supporting them every inch of their struggle...

The Nimpkish Band Council's submission demanded complete and autonomous control over all matters related to the delivery of health care to the Nimpkish Indian Band. This included the setting up of a Health Board which would co-ordinate all the relevant health, judicial and other social services, the hiring and firing of doctors, the implementation of training programs, etc. They reiterated the National Indian Brotherhood's position that good health and good health care could only be achieved by breaking the bonds of dependency on non-Indians and by placing these matters firmly under the control of Indian people themselves:

> You have heard from those Government officials whose responsibility it has been to provide medical services to Indians....They simply stood by as Indian people died. This evidence leads to only one conclusion. We cannot rely upon others to deliver health services to us....
>
> Some people may feel that our proposal for medical services designed around the central principle of Indian control will drive wedges rather than build bridges between Indian and non-Indian people in Alert Bay. This is not our intent. This proposal is designed to produce a first class health service which has built into it a responsiveness to the distinctive health needs of Indian people. Indian control should not be mistaken for a struggle for exclusivity but for excellence.

They also called for the removal of Dr. Harold Pickup:

> But Dr. Pickup remains a troubling stumbling block to our proposal. He personifies in the eyes of many Indian people the years in which Indian people have been subjected to second-class service. He symbolizes not the regaining but the taking away of our strength. We fear our proposal may not work, that we may not be able to develop the necessary commitment among our own people, that we may not be able to recruit the medical staff we need, that we may not be able to develop any working relationship between the Nimpkish Indian Health Centre and St. George's, if Dr. Harold Pickup remains in practice.

Dr. Goldthorpe spent twenty-three days in Alert Bay, several days in the surrounding villages and two weeks in Vancouver and Victoria. In May, 1980, he released his findings:[4]

> Despite its notoriety of the past year, the evidence of poor health, and health service problems, Alert Bay possesses a cultural fascination,

social warmth, and strengths in both its communities...

From countless hours of listening to residents of Alert Bay and surrounding communities, Indian and non-Indian, of discussions with present and former members of the hospital staff, with Dr. Pickup, with doctors who have worked with him, from study of written complaints against him submitted to the College of Physicians and Surgeons, and of the College's written responses, from study of hospital patient records and of reports and findings from inquests, I find:

(1) That Dr. Pickup possesses at least the minimum level of medical skill and knowledge to practice medicine in B.C., as found by the investigating committee of the College of Physicians and Surgeons in July, 1979; that is, he is competent, by that definition.

(2) That Renee Smith, and at least two other patients have died in St. George's Hospital as a result of Dr. Pickup's errors in judgment, or neglect.

(3) That the great majority of patients cared for in St. George's Hospital by Dr. Pickup have not had the benefit of a recorded medical history, physical examination, or progress note, during their hospital stay. This includes many patients who have died in hospital. This signifies inadequate medical care.

(4) That Dr. Pickup has been on many occasions clearly and obviously drunk while performing as a doctor in St. George's Hospital. That Dr. Pickup has been on many occasions clearly and obviously drunk in public in Alert Bay. That Dr. Pickup is an alcoholic in need of treatment.

(5) That hospital staff members of St. George's Hospital have complained in writing to the Hospital Board of Dr. Pickup's being drunk on duty and have received no reply, and have no knowledge of any resulting action by the Board.

That patients of Dr. Pickup, and staff members of St. George's Hospital, have complained in writing to the B.C. College of Physicians and Surgeons of Dr. Pickup's being drunk on duty in St. George's Hospital. The College has acknowledged receipt of the complaints and said it was referring some of the complaints to the committee investigating Dr. Pickup's competence. Other complaints it said it would investigate and communicate again with the complainant. However, the complainants received no further communication from the College.

That the B.C. College of Physicians and Surgeons acted inadequately and inappropriately in referring complaints of Dr. Pickup's drunkenness on duty and verbally abusive behaviour with patients, to the committee investigating Dr. Pickup's competence. Under the terms of Section 48A of the Medical Act,[5] that committee could consider only

Dr. Pickup's skill and knowledge, not his conduct or fitness to practise. The matters complained of were therefore outside the terms of reference of the committee, and it is not surprising that they were not referred to in the committee's findings. Similarly the questions raised of judgement and fitness to practice in the finding of negligence by the Renée Smith inquest could not be fully addressed by the investigating committee of the College.

The appropriate and adequate response of the College to the written complaints and the inquest findings would be to establish an Inquiry into Dr. Pickup's conduct and fitness to practise, under Section 49 of the Medical Act.[6] An appropriate action by the Council of the College on receipt of the findings of such an inquiry, would be to restrict Dr. Pickup's licence to practise, under Section 50 of the Medical Act,[7] with the conditions that he i) undertake a course of treatment for alcoholism, and, ii) practise only in a location where there is adequate peer review, that is, in a hospital with at least ten doctors on staff.

That the B.C. College of Physicians and Surgeons gives insufficient weight, in its consideration of complaints, to its duty to protect the public, and to protect the reputation of the profession, and gives excessive weight to protecting the interests of the physician complained about. It appears to require an unattainable amount of evidence before establishing an inquiry into fitness to practise, or conduct.

(7) That Dr. Pickup has been on many occasions verbally abusive, and disrespectful, toward Indian patients. It is not clear to me whether this represents racism. I do not know if on other occasions he has been abusive with non-Indian patients. I do know that many Indian patients continue to seek his care and to support him.

(8) That all agencies involved in these matters over the past year have privately urged Dr. Pickup to leave Alert Bay. At one time, Dr. Pickup had considered moving but changed his mind because he did not want to leave his patients without medical care. However I find it would be easier to recruit a long-term doctor to the village after Dr. Pickup leaves.

(9) That St. George's Hospital Board failed to fulfill its responsibilities in not suspending Dr. Pickup's hospital privileges...

From countless hours of discussion with St. George's Hospital Board and staff members, visits to the hospital, meeting patients, examination of Hospital Board minutes, hospital patient records, reports, and other relevant documents, I find:

(1) That the majority of patients admitted to St. George's Hospital do not require hospital care. They are being admitted by Dr. Pickup for their convenience or his or both. That patients are kept in hospital for periods beyond any medical need for hospitalization. This represents

an abuse of public facilities and funds.

(2) That the Hospital Board members have at least average motivation, knowledge and dedication to their responsibilities...However, the Board suffers a lack of sensitivity to Indian concerns and needs, and requires a great deal of support and assistance to be able to carry out its responsibility to monitor the quality of medical care in hospital, and to take appropriate action with medical staff.

Dr. Goldthorpe's report went on to lambast the government of the Province of B.C. for its lack of attention to Indian concerns, the Department of Fisheries and Oceans for poor management of salmon stocks and licensing procedures, and the Department of Indian Affairs for its relocation policies. However, when it came to his former employers, the federal Medical Services Branch/Indian Health Division, Dr. Goldthorpe was more sympathetic:

Several criticisms were leveled at Medical Services Branch during the Commission process. The strongest one charged the Medical Services failed to advocate strongly enough with appropriate authorities, in support of Indians it knew were getting inadequate care from Dr. Pickup and St. George's Hospital. The advocacy role is not an easy one for public servants...I find that Dr. Gordon Butler, as Regional Director, Pacific Region, Medical Services Branch, did carry out a reasonable advocacy function with regard to health care of Indians in Alert Bay, in a series of correspondence with the Registrar of the B.C. College of Physicians and Surgeons, after the death of Renee Smith in 1979. Former Medical Services public health nurse, Sandra Waarne, with tact and persistence in difficult circumstances, carried out an advocacy function with Dr. Pickup, on behalf of hospitalized Indians in need of referral to specialists, on her weekly ward rounds with him, for several years in the seventies. And Dr. Mary Habgood, most criticized in the matter, did confer with her supervisor for advice, did advise individual Indians to write to the B.C. College of Physicians and Surgeons, and did call the College herself. More cannot reasonably be expected of public servants, in the circumstances of sensitive relations among federal, provincial, and private institutions. ...I find that Zone Director, Dr. Habgood, is a caring and competent public servant, and recommend that no action be taken on the criticism of her before the Commission.

The second half of Dr. Goldthorpe's report was devoted to mortality statistics, and health in general among the Indian population of the Alert Bay area:

What a tragic waste of young life! 56% of Alert Bay Indians dead before age 40. For an Indian at birth, a 44% chance of reaching age 40. And for those not reaching 40 alive, alcohol or other drug abuse the major or contributing cause in 47 out of 74 or 63%. For those dying between 40 and 70, alcohol a major or contributing cause in 19 out of 40, almost half.

The Alert Bay Indian group had been experiencing 2.0 more deaths per thousand per year, or 5 more deaths per year for their entire population, than if the death rate for all Canadian Indians applied... In summary, then, from comparing death rates, Alert Bay Indians are less healthy than other B.C. Indians, and B.C. Indians are less healthy than other Canadian Indians. Since the crude death rates of Alert Bay Indians and of all Canadian Indians are 8.8 and 6.8, respectively, one can say that a Alert Bay Indian stands a 25% greater chance of dying within the next year than does an Indian elsewhere in Canada....

It is ironic, and probably not entirely coincidental, that those who had the most seem to have lost the most. B.C. was the most densely populated area in North America before white contact, richest in resources—fish, game, in leisure time, art, culture. Yet it came closest to being wiped out. Today the Alert Bay Indians, among the wealthiest and most sophisticated in Canada, suffer significantly higher death rates than Canadian Indians generally, and than the Ojibway and Cree of Northwestern Ontario, who speak little English and live in remote villages without running water or electricity or central heating.

There are other ways in which Alert Bay Indian health is poor, or worse than average for Indians in Canada:

-prematurity rate for last three years has been 11-14%

-75% of pregnancies are high risk

-respiratory infections are common

-anemia and nutrition problems and developmental delays are seen frequently

-six children were found with foetal alcohol syndrome in 1978

-infestations are common, head lice and scabies particularly

-[for] 1975-1979 nineteen cases of T.B. among fewer than 1000 Indians. This works out to 40/10,000/year as compared to 12.5/10,000/year for all Canadian Indians and 1.6/10,000/year for all Canadians.

-1978: 50 cases of hepatitis

-alcohol affects 90% of Alert Bay Indian families at one time or another.

Health has a less tangible dimension, not demonstrable by death or disease statistics, yet just as real and possibly more important. It is 'whole health', involving spiritual, social, and mental aspects of the life of the individual and the community. It is 'health as strength', as togetherness, as harmony with the universe, as self-esteem, pride in self and group, as self-reliance, as coping, as joy in living.

Their health has declined with suppression of their language and culture, with the anti-potlatch laws, with compulsory schooling away from home, family and language, with disrespect by powerful whites for their social and political institutions, with assimilationist assumptions that they should just join in general Canadian (or B.C.) social and political institutions, and forget their own. Their health has declined with the decline of salmon stocks, with the influx of welfare cheques. Their health has declined with the disappearance of communities where within living memory they were content and self-reliant.....This ill health is evident in loss of respect for self and others, for older people; in drinking to excess, fighting; in child neglect and apprehension, in suicide attempts. Generally it is fairly poor at present, this "subjective health", in Alert Bay Indians. Yet there is a ray of hope in the recognition of causes, and possibly the beginning of an upturn....

A significant change in the social and political environment of the community is needed. And the community has to be the Indian community, I have learned—cultural and political distance is too great between the two ends of Alert Bay, co-operation and compromise too minimal, for significant change to occur across the two communities all at once. A stronger, healthier Indian community should not threaten the people of the municipality, but should make Alert Bay a more attractive place for all to live.

Dr. Goldthorpe prescribed all sorts of cures for the many ills, ranging from financing a return to the deserted villages to the development of a terminal fishery at the river mouth and the construction of recreation facilities. He also recommended that Dr. Pickup move to a larger centre where he would be subject to more active peer review, that the B.C. Ministry of Health amend the Medical Act to allow the appointment of lay people to the Council of the B.C. College of Physicians and Surgeons and that the St. George's Hospital Society amend its constitution to increase Native representation. Dr. Goldthorpe agreed with the position taken by all the Native organizations and the Nimpkish Band that Native people should begin taking over the delivery of social services, education and health care within their own communities. He supported the band's proposal for the creation of a Nimpkish Indian Health Board to be made up of three salaried employees who would begin the necessary research and planning for the construction of a Nimpkish Indian Health Centre in which health and social services could be centralized, and a Health Home where alcoholics could detoxify, recuperate and receive on-going counselling.

An elated Nimpkish Band Council and Kwakiutl District Council and staff distributed Dr. Goldthorpe's report to the press. All their allegations against the doctor and the hospital had been vindicated—AGAIN!—and they were to take over their own health care.

Liberal Minister of Health Monique Begin had been returned to office in the recent federal election, and a meeting was immediately arranged among the Minister, her top officials and representatives of the Nimpkish Band Council and the Kwakiutl District Council, to discuss funding for the Health Board whose mandate would be to "pull together and co-ordinate all medical and social services for the purpose of providing a system of improved health care to Alert Bay and the surrounding villages."

A delegation led by chiefs and councillors, accompanied by Michael Jackson, flew to Ottawa to meet personally with the Minister and to sign the necessary contracts. The band and district councils declared victory!

The press, tired of Dr. Pickup stories, concentrated on the shocking statistics about alcoholism and mortality on the reserve, and the *Campbell River Upper Islander* editorialized:

> We shake our heads over the tragedies of history—from the Crucifixion to the Holocaust. But we have trouble recognizing the tragedies around us and even more difficulty mobilizing against them when they involve such subtle concepts as 'whole health.'
>
> A physician from Ontario has delivered a sensitive report after looking into the health and health services of Indians living at Alert Bay. It is not primarily the story of an alcoholic doctor working there or of a deficient hospital. It is first and foremost about a community state of mind.
>
> "Thriving Indian communities with their own social and political forms, perpetuating Indian culture...would be easier on the public purse than the present sad situation. They cannot be likened to apartheid because any Indian can leave freely to live elsewhere, and can leave with pride as an Indian," Dr. Goldthorpe said in an interview. Isn't that the reserve system, which has largely failed?
>
> Because Indian communities often failed to meet needs of the past does not mean they could not work now, with rekindled pride in culture and community and rational economic assistance from government. But only the Indians can make them work.
>
> The question is: are too many of them too sick to care?

Dr. Goldthorpe's recommendations were forwarded to all the relevant ministeries, associations and organizations mentioned in his report. The Hospital Board received a copy of the report and sent a letter to Dr. Goldthorpe protesting the fact that the 'so-called' public hearings had been held on the reserve, and that they had been expected to appear in the same room as a Band Council which was made up of "boors." They claimed that evidence presented at the

Inquiry was nothing but "emotional outbursts and hate-filled speeches." They went on to accuse the Band Council of being unrepresentative, and of being intent on dragging everyone into the abyss created by their "adventure in self-government" which was financed by Canadian taxpayers and which would not produce any "miraculous cure" for Indian youths' "natural inclination towards drug and alcohol abuse." All this was interspersed with references to the Parti Quebecois and Rene Levesque.

The Band Council didn't bother to reply.

The B.C. College of Physicians and Surgeons said that the kind of testimony presented at the Goldthorpe Inquiry would not constitute evidence at a College hearing into a doctor's competence. "We need more concrete evidence than the opinion of individual witnesses at specific occasions," Dr. Craig Arnold, College Registrar, told reporters.

The new Social Credit Minister of Health, Rafe Mair, said he had sent a telegram to Dr. Goldthorpe asking for further information so that appropriate action could be taken.

And a new Chief Coroner for B.C., Dr. William McArthur, told the press he was "stunned" by the report and commended Dr. Goldthorpe for his "thoroughness and diligence." Although he declined to make any direct comment on the Commissioner's findings, the coroner expressed his "strong support" for the recommendation that the public be represented in hearings of complaints against B.C. doctors.

Dr. Goldthorpe's report reflected his commitment to the concept of "whole health" as he had articulated it at the opening of the inquiry. The Department of National Health and Welfare, however, were the only ones obligated to officially respond to Dr. Goldthorpe's findings or recommendations, and they did so within the confines of their mandate and policy priorities. Since the federal government has no jurisdiction over either the St. George's Hospital Board, provincial hospitals, or the B.C. College of Physicians and Surgeons, the indignity of another public exposure was, in the long run, the only price paid by any of these agencies.

Their sun may have been setting but it still defined the horizon.

Dr. Pickup, who until now had refused to talk to the press, granted the reporter who had covered the Angela Richards inquest an interview—at the Legion—over rye and beer. The doctor was smug. He told the reporter, "my wife says you should not take pictures of me here in the Legion." But he allowed the photograph anyway.

Dr. Pickup held forth: "The radicals want me out so that they can take over health care up here even though they haven't got the competence to do it," he explained.

Nearly a full page in the *Vancouver Province* was devoted to this article which was supplemented by interviews with loyal Indian patients of Dr. Pickup's. The article continued:

> Dr. Pickup's only comment on what he earns from his practice is that his net income for 1979 was $60,000.00. On the basis of the $133,486.00 in gross payments to H. J. Pickup and Associates by the B.C. Medical Commission for the year ending March, 1979, he's among the highest-paid general practitioners in B.C.

Commissioner Goldthorpe left, and the media left, and the representatives of the provincial and federal governments left, and the Indian political organizations left. People in the community went back to living their lives.

Every day, everyone went down the road.

NOTES:

Sources for this chapter are: *The Goldthorpe Inquiry*, transcripts of proceedings, Vols. 1-III; tape recordings, newspaper reports and personal notes. The original sources have been edited to provide logical sequencing, to eliminate interruptions, repetitions and other inconsistencies, and for ease of reading.

[1]pseudonym

[2]pseudonym

[3]Relevant clauses of the *Medical Act of British Columbia*, Section 55: Duty To Report On Member, read as follows:

> (1) Every member registered under this Act shall report to the registrar the condition of any person registered under this Act whom he, on reasonable and probable grounds, believes to be suffering from a physical or mental ailment or emotional disturbance or addiction to alcohol or drugs, that, in his opinion, if he is permitted to continue to practise medicine or surgery, might constitute a danger to the public or be contrary to the public interest; and thereupon the registrar shall promptly report the matter to the executive committee, and the executive committee may suspend from practice the person so reported upon and shall promptly appoint an inquiry committee in accordance with subsection (2) of section 49 to investigate the matter and to report its findings to the Council; and the inquiry committee shall promptly examine the person so reported upon if he can be found within the Province, and consider such other evidence as it sees fit.
>
> (3) If the report of the committee is not to the effect that the person reported upon is fit to practise medicine or surgery, the Council or the executive committee may suspend from practice the person reported upon or, if the person has been suspended, his suspension shall continue.
>
> (7) If the committee is of the opinion that the applicant is fit to practise under certain restrictions, the executive committee may make an order accordingly under clause (c) of subsection (2) of section 50.

[4]These excerpts are summations of Canada, Government of, Commission on Indian Health in Alert Bay, B.C., Department of National Health and Welfare, Medical

Services/Indian Health Division (1980) Goldthorpe, Dr. G., Commissioner, *Report to the Minister of National Health and Welfare Canada.* The original source has been edited to provide logical sequencing and ease of reading.

[5]Relevant clauses of the *Medical Act of British Columbia*, Section 48(A): Investigations Into And Examinations of Skills, read as follows:

(1) The Council may at any time investigate in such manner as it sees fit whether or not a member of the College has and is bringing to his practice of medicine or surgery adequate skill and knowledge and may, for the same purpose, require such member to undergo such examinations as the Council may specify.

(2) If the Council, as a result of such investigation or examinations, is of the opinion that the member in question should not be permitted to practise or that his practice should be restricted, it may, as the case may be, act in accordance with clause (a) or clause (b) or clause (c) of subsection (2) of Section 50.

[6]Relevant clauses of the *Medical Act of British Columbia.* Section 49: Inquiry, read as follows:

(1) The Council or the executive committee may, and if it is requested in writing so to do by 3 members in good standing of the College shall, cause an inquiry to be made by an inquiry committee into any charge or complaint made against any member of the College or into a question concerning the conduct or mental condition or capability or fitness to practise of any member of the College. A charge or complaint need not be made in any particular form or manner and may originate with the Council or any committee of the Council.

(2) The Council or the executive committee causing an inquiry to be made under this section shall appoint any inquiry committee of not fewer than three from among the members of the Council or former members of the Council; but if in the opinion of the Council or the executive committee the charge, complaint, or question to be inquired into appears to concern the mental or emotional condition of a member of the College, the inquiry committee may consist of or include members of the College who are not members of the Council and shall include at least one psychiatrist.

(3) Notwithstanding anything contained in this section or Section 50, the Council or the Executive committee may cause the conduct of a member relating to his practice of medicine to be summarily investigated with a view to determining whether or not a complaint is frivolous or appears to be sufficiently serious to justify the appointment of an inquiry committee under this section. Where a complaint is found not to be frivolous but not sufficiently serious to justify the appointment of an inquiry committee, the Council may reprimand the member whose conduct was in question.

[7]Relevant clauses of the *Medical Act of British Columbia*, Section 50: Suspending or Erasing From Register, read as follows:

(1) An inquiry committee shall find the facts, and shall also find whether the charge or complaint (if any) has been proven, and shall report its findings to the Council in writing. At any time after it has commenced taking the evidence, respecting a charge or complaint, the inquiry committee may of its own motion suspend from practice the member whose conduct is under

inquiry until the next meeting of the Council and shall promptly give written notice of the suspension to the member and the registrar.

(2) If the Council upon a report made under subsection (1) considers that a member has been guilty of infamous or unprofessional conduct or that a member is incapable or unfit to practise, or that a member is suffering from a mental ailment, emotional disturbance, or addiction to alcohol or drugs that might, if the member continues to practise as a physician or surgeon, constitute a danger to the public, the Council may

(a) cause the name of the member to be erased from the register;

(b) suspend the member from practice for a period prescribed by the Council;

(c) cause the name of the member to be erased from the register or the temporary register under section 38 subject to whatever terms and conditions the Council may prescribe;

(d) impose on the member a fine not to exceed the sum of ten thousand dollars;

(e) reprimand the member; or

(f) suspend the imposition of punishment and place the member on probation upon whatever terms the Council may prescribe.

CHAPTER 12

Lessons From History

Alert Bay, B.C.
1895

Law and order came to the Alert Bay district when Mr. Philip Woollacott was stationed at Alert Bay as the first constable. He arranged to have some of the Indians themselves police their own reserves and they were sworn in as special constables. Some of them took their duties more seriously than was intended they should.

One of the settlers at Kingcome Inlet was a Mr. Baron Granville Blackwell,[1] a young Englishman from Bristol...

Early one morning Blackwell, who was a crack shot, heard a number of dogs barking near his place, and on going out found five dogs worrying some of his young cattle. He immediately opened fire, and killed three of the dogs. One got away, and one, the biggest of them all, though wounded, attempted to swim across the river. He died making the effort. His owner happened to discover the body floating in the stream, and, landing from his canoe at Blackwell's, he made enquiries. Mr. Blackwell told him that he had shot the dog and was only sorry that he had missed one and allowed it to escape. The Indian...returned to his village in high wrath.

Sensing trouble, Blackwell gathered his neighbours, and in a very short time two canoes laden with Indians showed up. Two of them informed the white settlers gathered there that they were Indian constables and showed their badges and handcuffs. They said they were going to take Mr. Blackwell to jail in Alert Bay...As they were obviously in an extremely vicious mood (and they had guns), Mr. Blackwell decided to go with them...

The Indians, true to their word, escorted Mr. Blackwell to Alert Bay...They could have easily murdered him in revenge for the loss of their dogs. Perhaps, however, they were aware of reprisals taken at different times by the British Navy and the Hudson's Bay Company when cannon loaded with grape shot had nearly wiped out Indian villages. As late as 1865, the HMS *Clio* destroyed a hostile village near Fort Rupert...

At any rate, Mr. Blackwell was brought safely to Alert Bay, where the Indians put him in irons and paraded him up and down as an example to the younger generation. Constable Woollacott, a man of good education and of good family from England, took an entirely different view of the matter than either of the two Indian constables, or Blackwell, had expected. He explained to the Indians that they could not arrest a man out of hand without a warrant. Woollacott then turned to Blackwell, and said to him:

"I thought you were an Englishman!"

"Well, I have that honour," Blackwell replied.

"You, an Englishman, allow yourself to be brought in here in this manner by untamed savages! I consider you a disgrace to the name of Englishman!" Woollacott bellowed, and then left to appeal to William Halliday, Magistrate, for the appropriate warrants. Halliday recalled the incident in his memoirs:

> I issued warrants against the two so-called policemen, and they were put under arrest, and to their intense surprise and chagrin, instead of their being the informants and plaintiffs, they became the defendants in the case. They were brought up for preliminary hearing on the charges of illegal arrest and abduction, and remanded for a week. At the end of the week they were again remanded for another week. As they acted in good faith and were absolutely sure they were in the right, they failed to understand their predicament.

Mr. Halliday pointed out to them that they had committed a grave offence by arresting a settler without a proper warrant, especially as their constabulary powers pertained only to the reserve. As the white people wished to live peacefully with the Indians at Kingcome Inlet, Mr. Blackwell would not press charges but would be satisfied if they were deposed from office as special constables and on the further condition that they would return him safely to his home. The Indians accepted this with very bad grace. They stated that the sight of Blackwell was an annoyance to them, and they absolutely refused to take him back with them to Kingcome Inlet in their canoe, but were willing to provide another canoe properly equipped in which he could have the privilege of rowing himself back again.

In the matter of keeping law and order among the Indians, very often harsh justice was meted out, but this was felt by those in authority to be the best means of teaching them the laws of the province which they now had to obey.

—from an account in: Halliday, William (1935) *Potlatch and Totem: Recollections of an Indian Agent*, J. M. Dent & Sons Ltd., Toronto, pp. 173-177, and *History of Alert Bay and District*, pp. 42-43.

NOTE:

[1]pseudonym.

Epilogue

After Dr. Goldthorpe's report was released those of us who had lived in the eye of the storm since Renee's death began trying, in various ways, to cope with the aftermath of the experiences we had been through. Some threw themselves into organizing the new Health Centre and trying to resolve the many conflicts within the community that the struggle had produced. Others continued the fight. Most picked up the pieces of their everyday lives and carried on. In June, 1980 my husband, myself, and our children, along with a few other members of the former Education Committee left Alert Bay to spend a few years in Vancouver. George and Kelly wanted to go to university; and I, feeling as though I'd been living in a house of mirrors, yearned for the familiar anonymity of the city. I had believed for a long time before moving to Alert Bay that the personal was political, but during the past year and a half I had come to understand that the political is personal, and I found this a difficult realization to come to terms with.

Alert Bay, B.C.
June, 1983

It is now four and a half years since Renee died and this year, 1983, is the 25th Anniversary of June Sports. A lot of work and planning has gone into the celebration, and the new Health Centre is scheduled to be officially opened on the weekend. Everyone who has come to visit us in Vancouver during the last few months has been really hepped up about both the Anniversary and the Health Centre. We discuss it and discuss it, coming to the conclusion that we can't afford either the time or the money to go, and besides it would mean Carey and Lori missing a week of school.

George leaves on the 16th with the kids, I finish some work and go up on the 19th.

OFFICIAL GRAND OPENING
OF THE NIMPKISH INDIAN HEALTH CENTRE

The Health Centre is a nice, modern cedar building, located behind the old residential school. There's a medical library and a reading room, a dental clinic, a conference room, and a series of offices. The offices are for a doctor whose income is to be subsidized, in part, by Indian Health/Medical Services; the Health Board Co-ordinator; Indian Health Nurse; Community Health Representatives; Social Development Workers; Youth Workers; Homemakers; a Probation Officer and several Alcohol and Drug Counsellors. There is a also going to be a "Health Home" which will be a halfway house for people to stay in when they first return to the community after taking alcohol treatment.

The chief and council and many of the old people are here, all dressed in button blankets. The room is packed with people, mostly local. A number of government officials are in the audience. Dr. Pickup, who is still practising, has been invited and is here with a young woman who someone tells me is his daughter, who has just graduated from medical school.

Speeches are made about new directions for our people, self reliance and a new hope for the future of our children. Bob Joseph, now D.I.A.N.D. District Manager for the Kwakwaka'wakw District, talks about how the Health Centre came to be. "Our people went through a lot of pain to get this building we are gathered in to-day," Bob tells the assembled guests. "It took a lot of strength and it took a lot of courage. There are some scars left from all that went on that aren't quite healed up yet. We should remember all those who helped us to get this whole thing started and who are not here with us to-day. We have lots of friends. We must remember our own people who are no longer with us."

No one says anything.

Wedledi Speck, now a member of the Kwakiutl District Council, begins his speech, staring directly at Dr. Pickup. "We should never forget that this whole movement towards better health would not have started if Renee's young life had not been stolen from her," Wedledi says solemnly.

No one says anything.

Tea and refreshments are served. The atmosphere is celebratory and triumphant.

Around 2:00 p.m. I am sitting on the field watching a soccer game when I see Debra get out of her car outside Mabel's place and I decide to go up there and b.s. with them for a while and see Debra's new baby. In Mabel's

270

kitchen, sitting around the table are her aunt, Susi; Susi's daughter, Connie; Debra's brother, Henry; Debra and Mabel.

Susi is eating herring eggs on kelp dipped in oolichan oil and she, Connie and Henry are working their way through a mickey of vodka. Susi is holding forth in her usual boisterous fashion about her in-laws and how they think their son is too good for her but if people knew what stories she could tell about *them*—if she wanted to be like that—they wouldn't be so quick to bad mouth *her*...

Everyone is laughing and teasing each other. The baby is gurgling happily while Debra, Mabel and I fuss over him. Susi keeps playfully hitting Henry on the arm, telling him, "Phone for me, Wees![1] Come on!"

Henry ignores these requests and finally turns to Susi and says "How come you keep touching me Susi? You tryin' to hustle me or something? I told you I don't like older women!"

Howls of laughter follow his comment.

"You cheeky little brat!" Susi gives Henry a slap—a real one this time, but keeps after him to phone. Henry works as a bookkeeper and so everyone expects him to do formal business for them. Finally he starts dialing. Henry grins at me when he picks up the phone.

"How're you feeling to-day, G'un? Can I order you something?" he teases. He gets someone on the line and says, "I'm calling for Susi Joe. She lost her pills. Can she talk to Dr. Pickup?" Then he passes the phone over to Susi.

Susi's voice changes to a childish, coy whine and she explains to Dr. Pickup how she lost her blood pressure pills and she's wondering if he could possibly phone the drug store and get her another prescription. She's speaking carefully, over-pronouncing her words in an effort to sound sober. She thanks the doctor profusely, hangs up and then starts in on Henry to phone a cab to pick up the pills at the drug store and deliver them to her on the soccer field where she is headed as soon as she finishes her drink.

Debra and I look at each other and roll our eyes. Then Debra tells me about getting her baby from the hospital.

"It was funny, you know, when I got to take baby home. Dr. Pickup was there when baby was discharged. When I was taking baby out of the hospital Pickup starts telling me 'you should bring him in for this shot and that shot...' I just looked at him, you know, 'cause he knows where I stand on things. So he says, real quick, 'Well, I mean, uh, uh, take him to the doctor of your choice, that is.' I just said 'Yeah, that's just exactly what I'm going to do!'"

"I really like the new doctor, he's been here quite a while now. Too bad he isn't staying. I went to see him and he told me all what to do with baby and everything and he lent me some books out of the library down at the Health Centre. It's a good library."

I spend the rest of the day on the field except for a few other visits to relatives. People are being exceptionally friendly. Mary tells me how glad she is that we came home for June Sports, how good everything is in the community now, and how everyone is working together. Melissa says, with a snort, after Mary leaves, "Yeah...everyone who *works* at the Health Centre thinks its great!"

After Melissa leaves I ask Linda about her comment. "Are people happy with the Health Centre, really?" I ask. "Does it make any difference?"

Linda thinks about it for a minute and then says, "Well, you know how it is...Everyone's got their gripes...But the way I look at it is, at least it's here. At least it's ours. And that's got to be better than the way it was before. It's a basis, you know. Like, maybe we have to get ourselves together and keep on top of it...But at least when we do, maybe we can change things we don't like. Maybe...I hope... I mean, damn it! After what people in this community went through to get it...it better be better!"

Other people who haven't really spoken to me voluntarily for years now are smiling and waving. People tell me that the band's school is thriving and its enrolment has increased substantially. The main problem it is facing now is securing funds for the large number of non-Indian students attending who have been attracted by the school's reputation for offering sound training in the basics, as opposed to the public school's looser approach to structure and discipline. There are lots and lots of people here. Wedledi tells me they've had to put extra ferries on for the last two days. He figures the population of the reserve has tripled for the weekend.

The soccer tournament is getting down to the finals and sides are firmly chosen. As usual, everyone—other than their loyal fans—wants anybody but the T-Birds to win, just because they always do and they think they're good, which they are. A couple of the teams from the outlying villages are giving the T-Birds a run for their money. Apparently the villages were really into getting their teams ready this year, the objective being to beat Alert Bay at the Anniversary Tournament.

In the bars the mood is good. Lots of fans try to out-cheer each other for their various teams but there aren't any fights. Laughing, teasing, bullshitting, insulting, laughing some more. It's an endless round.

On the way home we're picking our way along the dark road, climbing in and out of potholes, and talking about the weekend. George is naming off people who have come home whom he hasn't seen for years and years. We exchange bits of gossip. Did you see...did you hear about...

Taking a rest, I sit down by the side of the road.

"Is it just that I've been gone long enough that coming back for a big weekend like this makes it all seem so much better? Is it just nostalgia? Or are things any better?" I ask.

"I don't know. A bit of both, I guess. But this weekend is really special. I haven't seen everyone feeling this good for ages," George replies.

"This town drives me crazy," I say. "There's no reason for everyone to be feeling so good. Last winter was awful—85 per cent unemployment, everyone was on welfare. There's supposed to be a fishing strike this year. Two more boats got taken away. Pickup is still here. People are still ordering their drugs over the phone. The drinking is still as bad as ever...Nothing's changed, only some things have gotten worse..."

"That's not true that nothing's changed," George answers. "Things just haven't changed in the ways *you* think they should. The medical thing wasn't the first crisis this community has been through. It sure as hell isn't the last. What happened, happened—and everyone remembers...That's the trouble with you," he teases. "No sense of history!"

"Well," I grumble. "Still...there's no reason for people to be so cheerful."

"Sure there is," George laughs. "This is Alert Bay! It's June Sports! Everybody's home!"

NOTES:

[1] "Wees" is a Kwa'kwala term of endearment used to address a male of the same age or younger. "G'un" is the female equivalent.

Bibliography

Abbott, Donald N. (ed) (1981) *The World Is As Sharp As A Knife: An Anthology in Honour of Wilson Duff*. Victoria: British Columbia Provincial Museum.

Andersen, Doris (1982) *The Columbia Is Coming!* Sidney, B.C.: Gray's Publishing Ltd.

Armstrong, David (1980) *An Outline of Sociology as applied to Medicine*. Bristol: John Wright and Sons Ltd.

Asch, Michael (1984) *Home And Native Land, Aboriginal Rights and the Canadian Constitution*. Agincourt, Ontario: Methuen.

Ashworth, Mary (1979) *The Forces Which Shaped Them: A History of the Education of Minority Group Children in British Columbia*. Vancouver: New Star Books.

Braroe, Niels (1975) *Indian & White: Self-Image and Interaction in a Canadian Plains Community*. California: Stanford University Press.

Brody, Hugh (1975) *The People's Land*. Middlesex, England: Penguin Books.
_____ (1981) *Maps and Dreams*. Vancouver: Douglas & McIntyre.

British Columbia Hospital Insurance Service (1963) *Reference Material on the British Columbia Hospital Insurance Service, January 1949-January 1963*. Victoria: B.C. Hospital Insurance Service.

British Columbia Medical Association (1973) *Health Care Delivery in British Columbia*. Vancouver: BCMA.

British Columbia Social Planning and Review Council (1981) *Citizen's Guide to the Health Insurance System in B.C.: its history and present status*. Vancouver.

Burke, J. (1976) *Paper Tomahawks: From red tape to red power*. Winnipeg: Queenston House.

Canada, Government of (1980) *Indian Conditions: A survey*. Department of Indian and Northern Affairs, Ottawa.

Canada, Government of. Medical Services/Indian Health Division, *Annual Reports*, Department of National Health and Welfare, 1955-1982.

Canada, Government of. Commission on Indian Health in Alert Bay, Department of National Health and Welfare, Medical Services/Indian Health Division. (1980) transcript of proceedings, *In the Matter of an Inquiry into Health and Health Care in Alert Bay, B.C.*, Dr. G. Goldthorpe, Commissioner. Vols. I, II, III.

_____ (1980) Goldthorpe, Dr. G., Commissioner, *Report to the Minister of National Health and Welfare, Canada*

Canada, Government of. (1971) *Questions and Answers: The Federal Medical Care Program.* Ottawa: Department of National Health and Welfare.

Canada, National Council of Welfare (1982) *Medicare: the public good and private practice.* Ottawa.

Canadian Nurses Association (October 1978) *The Canadian Nurse,* Vol. 74, No. 9. Ottawa.

Cartwright, F.F. (1977) *A Social History of Medicine.* London: Longman.

Castellano, Marlene Brant (1982) "Indian Participation in Health Policy Development: Implications for Adult Education." *Canadian Journal of Native Studies,* Vol. 11, No. 1.

Charron, K. C. (1963) *Health Services, Health Insurance and their Inter-Relationship: A Study of Selected Countries.* Ottawa: Government of Canada, Department of National Health and Welfare.

Codere, Helen (1950) *Fighting With Property: A Study of Kwakiutl potlatching and Warfare, 1792-1930.* Seattle: University of Washington Press.

_____ (ed) (1966) *Kwakiutl Ethnography: Franz Boas.* Chicago: University of Chicago Press

Cohen, Anthony P. (1982) "Blockade: a case study of local consciousness in an extra-local event," in Cohen, Anthony P. (ed), *Belonging: Identity and Social Organization in British Rural Cultures.* Social and Economic Papers No. 11. Newfoundland: Institute of Social and Economic Research, Memorial University.

Cole, Douglas (1985) *Captured Heritage: The Scramble for Northwest Coast Artifacts.* Vancouver: Douglas & McIntyre.

Collison, William Henry (1981) *In the Wake of the War Canoe.* Sidney, B.C.: Sono Nis Press.

Curtis, Edward S. (1905) *The North American Indian,* Vol. 10. New York: Johnson Reprint Co.

Driben, P. and R. S. Trudeau (1983) *When Freedom is Lost: The Dark Side of the Relationship between Government and the Fort Hope Band.* Toronto: University of Toronto Press.

Drucker, P. (1965) *Cultures of the North Pacific Coast.* U.S.A.: Chandler Publishing.

Duff, Wilson (1965) *The Indian History of British Columbia, Vol. 1: The Impact of the White Man.* Victoria: Province of B.C., Ministry of the Provincial Secretary, Memoir No. 5.

Dunning, R. W. (1962) "Some Aspects of Governmental Indian Policy Administration," *Anthropologica,* 4(1).

_____ (1964) "Some Problems of Reserve Indian Communities: A Case Study," *Anthropologica,* 6(1).

Dyck, Noel (1979) "Powwow and the Expression of Community in Western Canada," *Ethnos,* 44(1-2).

_____ (1980) "Indian, Metis, Native: Some Implications of Special Status," *Canadian Ethnic Studies,* 12(1).

_____ (1981) "The Politics of Special Status: Indian Associations and the Administration of Indian Affairs," in Dahlie, J. and T. Fernando (eds) *Ethnicity, Power and Politics in Canada*. Toronto: Metheun.

_____ (1983)(a) "The Negotiation of Indian Treaties and Land Rights in Saskatchewan," in Nocolas, P. and M. Langton, *Aborigines, Land and Land Rights*. Canberra: Australian Institute of Aboriginal Studies.

_____ (1983)(b) "Representation and Leadership of a Provincial Indian Association," in Tanner, A. (ed) *The Politics of Indianness: Case Studies of Native Ethno-politics in Canada*, Social and Economic Papers No. 12. Newfoundland: Institute of Social and Economic Research, Memorial University.

_____ (ed) (1985) *Indigenous Peoples and the Nation-State*. Social and Economic Papers No. 14. Newfoundland: Institute of Social and Economic Research, Memorial University.

_____ (1986) "Negotiating the Indian 'Problem'," *Culture*, Vol. VI, No. 1.

Engels, F. (1969) *The Condition of the Working Class in England*. London: Panther.

Esland, G. and G. Salaman (eds)(1980) *The Politics of Work and Occupations*. Toronto: University of Toronto Press.

Fanon, Franz (1963) *Wretched of the Earth*. New York: Grove Press, Inc.

_____ (1963) *Black Skin, White Masks*. New York: Grove Press, Inc.

Fisher, Robin (1977) *Contact and Conflict: Indian-European Relations in British Columbia, 1774-1890*. Vancouver: University of British Columbia Press.

Ford, C. S. (1941) *Smoke From their Fires: The Life of a Kwakiutl Chief*. Connecticut: Archon Books, Yale University Press.

Foucault, Michel (1975) *The Birth of the Clinic*. New York: Random House.

Fry, Alan (1970) *How A People Die*. New York: Tower Publications Inc.

Gartrell, Beverley (1986) "'Colonialism' and the Fourth World: Notes on Variations in Colonial Situations," *Culture*, Vol. VI, No.1.

Gottschau, Walter (ed) (1979) Transcript: *Inquest into the Death of Renee Bernice Smith Held at the Alert Bay Coroner's Court*, April-June 1979, Vols. I & II.

Gusfield, Joseph R. (1975) *Community: A Critical Response*. New York: Harper & Row Publishers.

_____ (1981) *The Culture of Public Problems*. Chicago: University of Chicago Press.

Halliday, William (1935) *Potlatch and Totem: Memoirs of an Indian Agent*. Toronto: J. M. Dent & Sons Ltd.

Heagerty, J. J. (1940) *The Romance of Medicine in Canada*. Toronto: Ryerson Press.

Healey, Elizabeth (1958) *History of Alert Bay and District*, 1958 Alert Bay Centennial Committee. Comox: E. W. Bickle Ltd.

Illich, Ivan (1976) *Medical Nemesis: The Expropriation of Health*. New York:

Pantheon Books, Random House.

Jarvis, George K. and Menno Boldt (1982) "Death Styles Among Canada's Indians," *Social Science and Medicine* 16(14).

Johnson, Patrick (1983) *Native Children and the Child Welfare System.* Toronto: Canadian Council on Social Development and James Lorimer & Co.

Kennedy, Dorothy (1984) "The Quest For A Cure: A Case Study in the Use of Health Care Alternatives," *Culture,* IV (2).

Knight, Rolf, (1978) *Indians at Work: An Informal History of Native Indian Labour in British Columbia 1858-1930.* Vancouver: New Star Books.

_____ (1980) *A Man Of Our Times: Autobiography of a Japanese-Canadian Fisherman.* Vancouver: New Star Books.

Lambert, W. W. and W. E. Lambert (1964) *Social Psychology.* New Jersey: Prentice-Hall Inc.

Larsen, Sidsel Saugestad (1982) "The two sides of the house: identity and social organisation in Kilbroney, Northern Ireland," in Cohen, Anthony P. (ed) *Belonging: Identity and Social Organization in British Rural Cultures,* Social and Economic Papers No. 11, Newfoundland: Institute of Social and Economic Research, Memorial University.

_____, "Negotiating Identity: The Mic-Mac of Nova Scotia" in Tanner, A. (ed) *The Politics of Indianness: Case Studies of Native Ethnopolitics in Canada,* Social and Economic Papers No. 12. Newfoundland: Institute of Social and Economic Research, Memorial University.

LaRusic, I. et al (1979) *Negotiating a Way of Life: Initial Cree Experience with the administrative structures arising from the James Bay Agreement.* Montreal: SSDC Inc.

LaViolette, F. E (1973) *The Struggle for Survival: Indian Cultures and the Protestant Ethic in B.C.* Toronto: University of Toronto Press.

Lewin & Assoc., Inc. (1976) *Government Controls on the Health Care System: The Canadian Experience.* Washington, D.C.

_____ *Provincial Health Insurance Benefits.* Washington, D.C.

Lillard, Charles (1984) *Warriors of the North Pacific Coast.* Victoria: Sono Nis Press.

Little Bear, Leroy, M. Boldt and J. A. Long (eds) (1984) *Pathways to Self-Determination: Canadian Indians and the Canadian State.* Toronto: University of Toronto Press.

Loney, Martin (1977) "A political economy of citizen participation," in Panitch, L. (ed) *The Canadian State: Political Economy and Political Power.* Toronto: University of Toronto Press.

MacPherson, C.B. (1965) "Old and New Dimensions of Democracy," *The Real World of Democracy*, Massey Lectures, 4th Series. Canadian Broadcasting Corporation.

Mahon, Rianne (1977) "Canadian public policy: the unequal structure of representation," in Panitch, L. (ed) *The Canadian State: Political Economy and Political Power*. Toronto: University of Toronto Press.

Mauss, Marcel (1954) *The Gift*. London: Routledge & Kegan Paul.

McKenchie, Robert E. II (1972) *Strong Medicine: History of Healing on the North-West Coast*. Vancouver: J. J. Douglas.

McKinlay, John B. (ed) (1984) *Issues in the Political Economy of Health Care*. New York: Tavistock Publications.

Mills, C. W. (1959) *The Sociological Imagination*. New York: Oxford University Press.

Morgan, L. H. (1877) *Ancient Society*. New York: Henry Holt and Company.

Paine, Robert (ed) (1977) *The White Arctic: Anthropological Essays in Tutelage and Ethnicity*. Newfoundland: Institute of Social and Economic Research, Memorial University.

_____, *Patrons and Brokers in the Eastern Arctic*. Social and Economic Papers No. 2, Newfoundland: Institute of Social and Economic Research, Memorial University.

Panitch, Leo (1977) "The role and nature of the Canadian state," in Panitch, L. (ed), *The Canadian State: Political Economy and Political Power*. Toronto: University of Toronto Press.

Province of British Columbia, Ministry of Health (1978) *B.C.M.S.C. Payment Schedule*.

Robertson, Heather (1970) *Reservations Are For Indians*. Toronto: James Lewis & Samuel.

Rohner, Ronald P. (1967) *The People of Gilford: A Contemporary Kwakiutl Village*. Ottawa: National Museum of Canada, Bulletin No. 225.

Rosaldo, Renato, (1980) "Doing Oral History," *Social Analysis*, No. 4.

Rose, T. F. (1972) *From Shaman to Modern Medicine: A Century of the Healing Arts in British Columbia*. Vancouver: Mitchell Press.

Ryan, E. B. and H. Giles (eds) (1982) *Attitudes towards Language Variation*. London: Edward Arnold.

Schwimmer, E. G. (1972) "Symbolic Competition," *Anthropologica*, 14(2).

Sewid-Smith, Daisy (1979) *Prosecution of Persecution*, Nu-Yum-Balees Society, Comox: E. W. Bickle Ltd.

Shortt, S. E. D. (ed) (1981) *Medicine in Canadian Society: Historical Perspectives*. Montreal: McGill-Queen's University Press.

Speck, George Jr. unpublished field notes, 1983-84.

Spradley, James P. (ed) (1969) *Guests Never Leave Hungry: The Autobiography of James Sewid, a Kwakiutl Indian*. New Haven: Yale University Press.

_____ (1980) *Participant Observation*. U.S.A.: Holt, Rinehart & Winston.

Stanbury, William T. (1975) *Success and Failure: Indians in Urban Society*. Vancouver: University of British Columbia Press.

Staum, M. S. and D. E. Larsen (eds) (1981) *Doctors, Patients and Society: Power and Authority in Medical Care*. Waterloo: Wilfred Laurier University Press.

279

Stearns, Mary Lee (1981) *Haida Culture in Custody: The Masset Band.* Vancouver: Douglas & McIntyre.

Swartz, Donald (1977) "The politics of reform: conflict and accommodation in Canadian health policy," in Panitch, L. (ed), *The Canadian State: Political Economy and Political Power.* Toronto: University of Toronto Press.

Tanner, A. (ed) (1983) *The Politics of Indianness: Case Studies of Native Ethnopolitics in Canada.* Social and Economic Papers No. 12. Newfoundland: Institute of Social and Economic Research, Memorial University.

_____ (1983) "Canadian Indians and the Politics of Dependency," in Tanner, A. (ed) *The Politics of Indianness, Case Studies of Native Ethnopolitics in Canada,* Social and Economic Papers No. 12. Newfoundland: Institute of Social and Economic Research, Memorial University.

Tennant, Paul (1982) "Native Indian Political Organizations in British Columbia, 1900-1969: A Response to Internal Colonialism," *B.C. Studies,* 55.

_____ (1983) "Native Indian Political Activity in British Columbia, 1969 - 1981," *B.C. Studies,* 57.

Thompson, E.P. (1966) *The Making of the English Working Class.* New York: Vintage Books.

Tobias, John L., (1983) "Protection, Civilization, Assimilation: An Outline History of Canada's Indian Policy," in Getty, Ian A. L. and Antoine S. Lussier (eds), *As Long as the Sun Shines and Water Flows. A Reader in Canadian Native Studies.* Vancouver: University of British Columbia Press.

Tolmie, William Fraser (1963) *Physician and Fur Trader.* Vancouver: Mitchell Press.

United Fishermen & Allied Workers Union (1971) *A Ripple, A Wave: History of trade union organizing in the west coast fishing industry.* Vancouver: Trade Union Research Bureau.

Ward, Peter W. (1981) "Class and Race in the Social Structure of British Columbia, 1870 - 1939," in Peter W. Ward and Robert A. J. McDonald (eds), *British Columbia: Historical Readings.* Vancouver: Douglas & McIntyre.

Weaver, Sally M. (1981) *Making Canadian Indian Policy: The Hidden Agenda 1968-1970.* Toronto: University of Toronto Press.

Wellman, David T. (1977) *Portraits of White Racism.* Cambridge : Cambridge University Press.

Wike, Joyce (1951) *Effect of the Maritime Fur Trade on Northwest Coast Indian Society,* Ph.D. dissertation, New York: Columbia University.

Wilson, Elizabeth (1977) *Women and the Welfare State.* London: Tavistock.

Wilson, J. (1977) "Social Protest and Social Control," *Social Problems,* 24.

Wolcott, Harry F. (1964), *A Kwakiutl Village and Its School: Cultural Barriers to Classroom Performance.* California: Stanford University Press.

Wolf, Eric (1982) *Europe and the People Without History.* Berkeley: University of California Press.